OVERCOMING DEPRESSION

Diagnosis & Treatments

2013 Report

A Special Report published by the editors of
Mind, Mood & Memory
in conjunction with
Massachusetts General Hospital
Boston, Massachusetts

Overcoming Depression: Common Problems & Treatments

Consulting Editor: Jonathan E. Alpert, MD, PhD, Associate Chief of Psychiatry and Associate Director, Depression Clinical and Research Program, Massachusetts General Hospital, and Joyce R. Tedlow, Associate Professor of Psychiatry, Harvard Medical School

Author: Alison Palkhivala

Group Directors, Belvoir Media Group: Diane Muhlfeld, Jay Roland

Creative Director, Belvoir Media Group: Judi Crouse

Associate Editor, Belvoir Media Group: Kristine Lang

Production: Darbi Bossman

Publisher, Belvoir Media Group: Timothy H. Cole

ISBN: 1-879620-92-8

To order additional copies of this report or for customer service questions, please call 877-300-0253, or write to Health Special Reports, 800 Connecticut Avenue, Norwalk, CT 06854-1631.

2013

Report on Overcoming Depression
Diagnosis & Treatments

You can't see depression. It doesn't cause a fever or rash. Doctors can't diagnose it using images of the brain or with blood tests (although one day that might be possible). In part because the symptoms of depression can be hard to separate from normal emotions or behaviors, and in part because of the stigma still associated with it, depression often goes undetected and undiagnosed.

Those who have never experienced depression sometimes find it hard to take seriously. They may be unable or unwilling to understand why their depressed family members or friends can't just pull themselves out of their funk. Anyone who has experienced depression knows exactly why they can't just "snap out of it." They've experienced the numbing fatigue, the ravaged self-esteem and the desire to do nothing but curl up in bed and pull the covers over their head. They know how significantly depression affects their relationships, work and virtually every other aspect of their lives.

Getting treatment for depression isn't as simple as popping a few pills. It's not an infection that will clear up in days or weeks. It can take months or sometimes years of treatment, often punctuated by relapses and setbacks, to finally achieve good control of depression.

Yet depression can be effectively treated, and people who have lived in its shadow can step back into the light and begin to enjoy life once again. Treatments for depression have come a long way over the last few decades. Now there are medications with fewer side effects than before, along with other therapies that directly target the parts of the brain that contribute to depression.

In this report, you'll learn about the latest research on depression, and you'll discover new therapies that are changing the lives of people around the world. You will also learn how to identify whether you or a loved one has depression, and the best places to turn for treatment and support.

■ ■ ■

HIGHLIGHTS

TABLE OF CONTENTS

Overcoming Depression
Diagnosis and Treatments
2013 Report

INTRODUCTION

Have you ever had one of those days? You know, the kind of day where everything seems to go wrong? After sitting in traffic, getting yelled at by your boss and burning dinner, you're ready to throw in the towel. You feel miserable about yourself, your life and the world in general. By the next day, though, your spirits are back up and the world starts looking like a brighter place again.

But what if you don't feel better the next day? What if, instead of rebounding from a hard day, you just slip further and further into misery and negative thinking? And what if that misery lasts not for hours or even days, but for weeks and months and affects your sleep, appetite, concentration, energy and ability to enjoy the things you once loved? When you have dark feelings that last for more than a couple of weeks and interfere with your daily life, and there is no obvious cause such as the recent death of a loved one, you may have depression.

If you or a loved one is feeling depressed, it is important for you to know that you are far from alone—depression affects about 121 million people on the planet, according to the World Health Organization. In fact, depression is one of the leading causes of disability worldwide.

According to the National Institute for Mental Health, nearly 7 percent of adults in the U.S. are depressed during any given 12-month period, and 2 percent would qualify as severely depressed. At any given time, about 3 to 5 percent of Americans are experiencing major depression, and just over 15 percent will experience major depression at some point during their lifetime. This burden of illness has its costs, and these affect everyone. Every year in the U.S., lack of production due to depression costs the economy more than 31 billion dollars.

Depression is not a sign of emotional weakness. It is a medical condition—just like diabetes or heart disease—and it can have serious, long-lasting repercussions on your work, relationships and health. Depression can disrupt your sleep, lower your self-esteem and even change your personality, making you more withdrawn, irritable or thin-skinned. It can make you more likely to smoke cigarettes and abuse alcohol and drugs. When left untreated, depression can even lead to suicide. In the year 2000, suicide claimed nearly one million lives around the world, and 10 to 20 times as many people attempted suicide. Suicide is among the top 20 causes of death overall and among the top three for individuals aged 15 to 34.

Fortunately, a number of therapies are highly effective at relieving the symptoms of depression and suicidal thoughts. Medication, talk therapy (psychotherapy), certain device-based therapies and a variety of natural complementary and alternative remedies can lift the blanket of misery and help you get back to being yourself again. Every day, researchers are learning a little bit more about what causes depression, and what they are learning is helping them develop newer, even more effective treatments.

The first step in getting help is recognizing that you have depression. Use this report as a guide to learn the symptoms and signs and compare them to what you (or a friend or loved one) are experiencing. Then, read about the various treatments available and discuss them with your doctor to find the therapy (or combination of therapies) that is best for you. Learn where to get help when you need it, so you can start feeling better and reclaim your life. ■

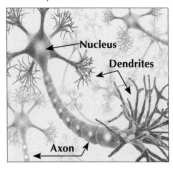
1 CAUSES OF DEPRESSION

For years, people with depression were told, "It's all in your head." That may be true in that it is a medical condition that affects your brain, but it doesn't mean it's in your imagination. It doesn't stem from out-of-control emotions or weakness, either. Depression is caused by a combination of genetic, environmental, biochemical and psychological factors.

How The Brain Regulates Mood

To understand what is happening in your brain when you have depression, it's helpful to understand how your brain works. Though it weighs only about three pounds and makes up just 2 percent of your body, your brain is a highly sophisticated piece of machinery. It has to regulate and coordinate all of the complex functions needed to keep you alive (i.e., breathing, heart rate, temperature regulation), and control your interactions with your environment (i.e., walking, talking, seeing, hearing, reasoning and feeling emotions).

BOX 1-2: MESSAGE PASSING ACROSS A SYNAPSE

Neurotransmitters pass across the synapses between nerve cells, enabling these cells to communicate.

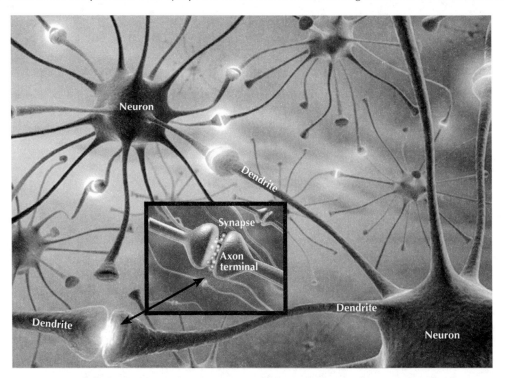

To accomplish all of these tasks, your brain is designed like a super-fast computer. It is wired with a network of interconnected nerve cells, called neurons. One hundred billion of these nerve cells transmit messages instantaneously throughout your brain and to the rest of your body (Box 1-1). Each of these neurons is so tiny that you could fit 50 of them side-by-side inside the dot at the top of this "i."

Messages speed from one neuron to another through branching projections called dendrites. Nerve messages are both electrical and chemical. First, an electrical signal travels through the neuron cell body to the axon at its end (called the axon terminal). At the very end is a tiny gap between the first neuron and the dendrite on the second neuron. This gap is called a synapse. When the electrical signal reaches the axon terminal, chemical messengers called neurotransmitters from the first neuron pass across the synapse to a receptor on the dendrite of the receiving neuron (Box 1-2).

Now, let's take a look at the brain as a whole. The brain is made up of several parts, each of which controls different functions (Box 1-3). Making up the bulk of the brain (85 percent) is the cerebrum, which controls thinking,

BOX 1-3: THE BRAIN

Different parts of the brain are responsible for different aspects of thought, mood and behavior. For example, the frontal lobe is responsible for speech, emotion, behavior, movement, intellect and planning, while the temporal lobe handles personality, memory and language.

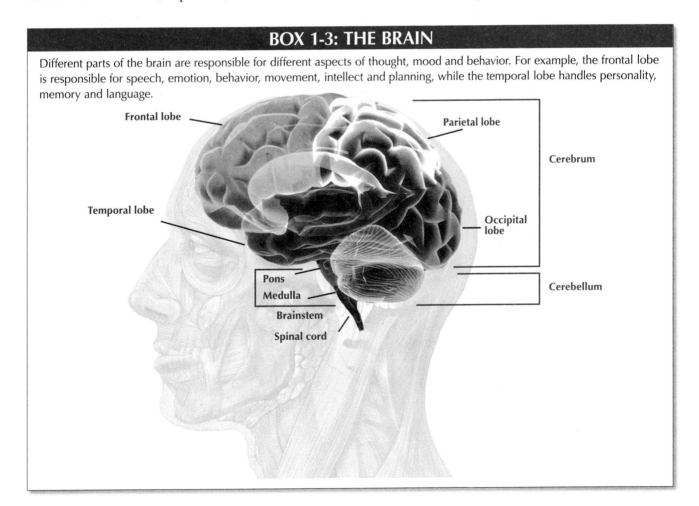

Frontal lobe

Parietal lobe

Cerebrum

Temporal lobe

Occipital lobe

Pons

Medulla

Cerebellum

Brainstem

Spinal cord

intellect, long- and short-term memory and motor function. You use this part of the brain when you balance your checkbook, or when you realize that you'd better buy extra chicken because you just remembered that your friends are coming over for dinner tonight. Next is the cerebellum, which is only one-eighth the size of the cerebrum but is no less important. It's in charge of balance and coordination. The brain stem connects the brain with the spinal cord, keeping you alive by regulating crucial body functions like breathing, digestion and blood circulation.

If you compare the brain of someone with depression to the brain of someone who is not depressed, on the outside they look pretty similar. However, when imaging scans such as magnetic resonance imaging (MRI) have been used to look inside the brain, discernible differences have been noted in the brains of people with depression, particularly with long-term or chronic depression that has persisted over years (Box 1-4).

People with a history of chronic depression have been found, on average, to have a smaller hippocampus—a part of the brain that is involved in memory—and a thinner right cortex, which is involved in mood. Researchers still don't know the exact reasons for these differences, but they may reflect the long-term impact on the brain of biochemical changes related to stress and depression. In turn, these differences may

BOX 1-4: BRAIN SCAN

Brain scans clearly illustrate reduced brain activity in people with depression. (Lighter areas represent brain activity.)

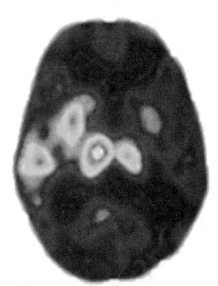

Reduced brain activity
in person suffering
from depression

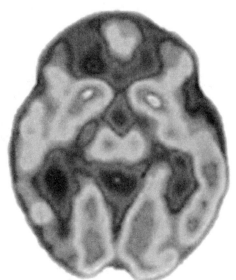

Normal brain activity
in person who doesn't
have depression.

affect the brain's ability to process emotional stimuli and respond to new environmental stresses.

Normal activity in the brain is also disrupted in depression. Regions of the brain that are involved in reward processing are less active in depressed people. As a result, people who are depressed sometimes say that they have almost entirely lost the experience of pleasure (a symptom called *anhedonia*). Many people with depression no longer look forward to activities they once enjoyed, like traveling to a favorite destination, watching a favorite sport or going out with friends.

You might have heard that depression stems from a "chemical imbalance," and that is partly true. In people with depression, the levels of certain brain chemicals are thought to be out of balance, particularly the neurotransmitters serotonin (which regulates mood, emotion and sleep), dopamine (which affects movement, attention and feelings of pleasure) and norepinephrine (which regulates arousal, sleep, attention and mood). Antidepressant medications are believed to work, in part, by helping correct these brain chemical imbalances.

In addition, other brain chemicals are likely to be involved in the signs and symptoms of depression. In recent years, attention has focused on the neurotransmitter glutamate, brain-derived neutrotrophic factor (BDNF), and other naturally occurring nerve growth factors in the nervous system. Stress and immune markers, such as corticotrophin releasing hormone (CRH) and inflammatory cytokines, may also play roles. These discoveries have raised the possibility of new treatments for depression that act on chemicals other than serotonin, norepinephrine and dopamine, which current medications target.

The more researchers study the brains of depressed people, the more they are able to pinpoint specific brain abnormalities associated with each aspect of depression. Several research projects conducted in 2012, for instance, have linked specific features of depression, including disrupted or unbalanced feelings of guilt, the tendency to ruminate about negative thoughts, anhedonia and disruptions in memory, with very specific brain imbalances or abnormalities.

What Causes Depression?

The brain plays an important part in depression, but it's not the only factor involved. Although your brain's design might predispose you to depression, typically other factors—such as stress, genes or illness—must exist for you to actually become depressed. Let's look at some of the other factors that can lead to depression:

Stress

Whether we like it or not, stress is a big and ongoing part of life. We face constant pressures—to succeed at work, to support our families, to meet the expectations set for us by our loved ones, friends and co-workers. Stress, in appropriate amounts, is actually a good thing. Without it, we wouldn't even bother to get up in the morning. But the key is balance. Just as too little stress leaves us without motivation to do anything, too much for too long can wear us out and lead to illness.

Here's why long-term stress is so detrimental. Say you're doing a little shopping at the mall. As you walk back to your car in the parking garage, you notice someone behind you. He seems to be following you. There's no one else in the garage, and you're still far away from your car. Your body goes into an alarm mode commonly called the "fight-or-flight" response. Your brain sends out an alert to the HPA axis— the hypothalamus, pituitary gland and adrenal glands. These glands release hormones such as adrenaline and cortisol, which surge through your bloodstream, speeding your heart rate and breathing and sending energy rushing to muscles and other areas of your body where it is needed most. This response is preparing you to either fight or run. The "fight-or-flight" response is very helpful when you're in immediate danger, but when it fires continually and over the long term it can be damaging to your health.

Those stress hormones are part of the reason why the stress that children experience in childhood can stay with them throughout their lives, increasing their risk for anxiety and depression in adulthood. A previous study found that adults who were abused or mistreated as children have higher levels of inflammatory blood markers such as cytokines or interleukin-6 in response to stress. These markers have been linked to depression and anxiety disorders.

Researchers have also found that the HPA axis is overactive in some people who are depressed. Having an excess of stress hormones can disrupt your brain's natural chemistry. Results from animal studies suggest that constant exposure to stress hormones damages brain cells, making your brain less able to regulate the stress hormone response.

Stress can also lead to depression and other illnesses by keeping your mind so preoccupied that it is unable to focus on activities that maintain your health. When you're stressed out, it's easy to forget to eat healthy and exercise. It's also easy to slip into bad habits like drinking and smoking cigarettes.

So, we know that stress has a big influence on depression. But why is it that some people can handle a lot of stress and never experience depression, while others fall apart at the slightest bit of stress? The answer to that and other questions about depression may lie in our genes.

It's In Your Genes

Researchers know that some people are more susceptible to depression than others. Now, thanks to genetic research, they are discovering why. In 2003, one group of researchers linked a variant of the serotonin transporter gene (5-HTT) with an increased risk of developing depression following stressful experiences. In 2011, researchers at the University of Michigan conducted an exhaustive review of 54 studies that included nearly 41,000 participants, and their findings seem to confirm that a person's genetic make-up has a significant impact on how he or she responds to stress.

Recently, researchers have honed in on several additional genetic variants that may help trigger depression and which may eventually provide new targets for depression treatment (Box 1-5). Scientists have also pinpointed five gene variants that may increase the likelihood that someone with depression will try to commit suicide. The variants are related to the survival, growth and connectivity of neurons. People with three of these mutations are nearly five times more likely to attempt suicide.

Genetic variants are likely why members of some families are more prone to mental illness than others, or why identical twins (who not only look the same but who have very similar DNA) are more likely to share depression than fraternal twins or siblings. Genes might also play a role in determining how well a person responds to antidepressant medications. Although genetic and other laboratory tests cannot yet determine which antidepressant medication will work best for a given person, progress is being made toward the development of this type of test, which will undoubtedly help guide treatment in the future.

Box 1-5: Depression susceptibility genes could provide new targets for treatment

Scientists are honing in on genes that increase a person's likelihood of developing depression. These genes may provide new targets for depression therapy in the future.

Over the past several years, a gene known as 5-HTTLPR has been repeatedly linked to depression in research studies. This gene influences the receptor for the neurotransmitter serotonin, which plays a key role in the regulation of emotion. Depression is a complex disease, however, and it's clear that no one gene explains the whole picture for everyone. Ongoing research continues to identify new candidate genes that are involved in depression.

For instance, in the April 28, 2011 issue of *Neuron*, researchers announced that they had discovered a link between depression and a gene known as SLC6A15. People with under functioning variants of this gene are at greater risk for major depression. Thus, these gene variants could become targets for new, more focused therapies for depression.

In another study published in the January 2012 issue of *Biological Psychiatry*, researchers combined all the types of information that have been previously linked with depression—including questionnaires, brain characteristics and behaviors—and looked for a single gene that could help explain the "whole picture" of depression. They found a potential candidate in RNF123. While this gene has not been previously linked with depression, it is known to affect the hippocampus of the brain, and alterations in the hippocampus have been implicated in depression.

Genes are important, but just because your mother and sister were depressed it doesn't mean that you are destined to follow the same path. Genes are just one part of the depression equation. Environmental influences are also important—including certain illnesses.

Illness

When your body feels miserable, your mind often follows suit. Anyone who has ever had the flu knows how down in the dumps you can feel when you're stuck in bed all day, unable to do anything but cough and blow your nose. Now imagine being sick not for days, but for months or even years.

It's no surprise that depression is common among people with chronic illnesses—particularly among those with debilitating conditions like chronic pain, cancer, diabetes or heart disease. For example, about one-third of stroke survivors develop depression, and one in five people hospitalized for a heart attack experience major depression. There are probably multiple reasons why depression is a frequent complication of chronic illness. Pain as well as loss of function and independence associated with certain chronic conditions can lead to demoralization and eventually depression. Certain chronic conditions, like stroke, Parkinson's disease or multiple sclerosis, affect brain regions that control mood and behavior.

But the relationship between illness and depression is actually a two-way street. That is, depressed people are more likely to suffer from chronic illnesses such as heart disease, and they also have a poorer prognosis than those without depression who have the same illness (Box 1-6).

These findings help explain the results of other studies, such as one published in the November 2011 issue of the *Archives of General Psychiatry*, which suggests that depression or a history of attempted suicide among individuals under the age of 40 markedly increases the risk of dying from heart disease later in life. The association was particularly strong in women, for whom depression was linked with fourteen times the risk of dying from a heart attack. In other research, depression was linked with a 45 percent increased risk for stroke. Both depression and chronic stress have also been linked with accelerated aging and an increased risk of developing dementia later in life.

In addition to the finding that chronic inflammation may underlie both depression and medical illnesses later in life, it is also recognized that depression increases the risk of medical illness and worsens its prognosis in other ways. In particular, depression frequently interferes with the motivation and ability to take good care of oneself. Depressed individuals are less likely to adhere to a healthy diet and a regular exercise regimen, are more likely to smoke and drink and are less likely to follow-up with medical evaluations and treatments.

Many people who are chronically ill don't realize that they're depressed or seek help for their depression because they assume it's natural to feel down during a long illness. Sometimes even loved ones, physicians and other caregivers will adopt the view that depression is "normal" in someone who is dealing with a chronic medical illness. It's true that depression is often related to the pain or incapacity of having an illness, but just because depression is one of the complications of having a general medical illness, there is no reason to let it continue. Just as you treat the symptoms of your illness, you should also treat the depression that occurs with that illness. Indeed, because depression can affect self-care and the prognosis of other medical illnesses, treating the depression that occurs with a general medical illness is often crucial to treating both.

Lifestyle

Lifestyle can play a significant role in the risk of becoming depressed. Lifestyle can also help explain the link between depression and other chronic illnesses, since the same negative lifestyle factors that can make you prone to depression also negatively affect other aspects of health.

Several studies have linked poor diet with an increased risk of depression. But it's not all about your diet. Research published in the online journal *PLoS ONE* in 2012 linked overworking with a twofold increase in the likelihood of depression.

The relationship between a lack of physical activity and depression also has been fairly well established. For instance, research from the November 2011 issue of the *American Journal of Epidemiology* linked less exercise and more time spent in front of the television with higher depression rates among women. On the plus side, exercise has been shown to help alleviate depression.

The relationship between lifestyle and depression is a chicken-and-egg one. That is, poor lifestyle habits can lead to depression, and depressed people frequently slip into poor lifestyle habits. When you can barely drag yourself out of bed, it can be unimaginably difficult to exercise or cook yourself a healthy meal.

Drugs

As mentioned above, another reason for the high prevalence of depression among people with medical illnesses is the medications used to treat those illnesses. Certain medications affect the levels of serotonin and other brain chemicals. Other drugs are very sedating. They slow down thinking, making people feel sleepy, withdrawn and unmotivated.

See Box 1-7 for a list of some medications that can cause depression. If you're taking one of the medications listed, and you are feeling unusually sad or withdrawn or you are having suicidal thoughts, talk to your doctor right away. You may need to change the dose or switch to another drug.

It's not only prescribed drugs that have been linked with depression. Use of several illicit drugs has also been shown to increase susceptibility to the disease. Abuse of amphetamines (commonly known as "speed") and MDMA ("ecstasy" or "E") in adolescence has been shown to increase the risk of depression later in life by 60 to 70 percent. Amphetamines in particular have been shown at high doses to permanently alter brain activity associated with the key neurotransmitters serotonin, dopamine and norepinephrine, which may explain why the drug increases the risk for depression.

BOX 1-7: MEDICATIONS THAT CAN CAUSE DEPRESSION		
DRUG	COMMON NAMES	COMMON USE
Alcohol	Beer, wine, spirits	Relaxation, socializing
Anticonvulsants	Zarontin, Topiramate	Treat epileptic seizures
Barbiturates	Phenobarbital, Secobarbital	Sedatives
Benzodiazepines	Librium, Valium	Treat anxiety, insomnia
Beta-adrenergic blockers	Lopressor, Inderal	Treat high blood pressure, heart problems
Calcium-channel blockers	Cardizem, Procardia	Treat high blood pressure, heart problems
Birth control medications	Norplant, some oral contraceptives	Prevent pregnancy
Corticosteroids	Prednisone	Treat arthritis and other inflammatory diseases
Fluoroquinolone antibiotics	Cipro, Floxin	Treat bacterial infections
Interferon alpha	Intron A, Roferon-A	Treat hepatitis B, certain cancers
Isotretinoin	Accutane	Treat acne
Opioids (narcotics)	Codeine, Demerol, OxyContin	Pain relievers
Statins	Zocor, Prevachol, Lipitor	Lower cholesterol
Varencline	Chantix	Smoking cessation

Among those who are genetically vulnerable to depression, smoking cannabis (e.g., marijuana, hashish) during adolescence also increases the risk of becoming depressed later in life.

The association between illicit drug use and depression may also be a bit of a chicken-and-egg conundrum because depressed people may be tempted to self-medicate with illicit drugs. Researchers out of Duke University have shown that treating major depression in adolescence with antidepressant medication reduces the likelihood that these adolescents will abuse drugs.

Hormones

Hormones are chemical messengers produced by the glands of the endocrine system that regulate various functions throughout the body. The release of hormones is governed by a very sensitive feedback system, which is controlled by the hypothalamus and pituitary gland in the brain. When hormones are produced in excess or in too limited of a supply, certain body functions won't work as well as they should. Depression is one of the potential side effects of a hormonal imbalance.

The butterfly-shaped thyroid gland in the neck produces hormones that regulate growth, metabolism and mood. When this gland is underactive (hypothyroidism) or overactive (hyperthyroidism), one of the symptoms may be depression. Disorders of the parathyroid glands (hyperparathyroidism) and adrenal glands (Cushing's disease) can also lead to depression.

Hormone shifts are one of the reasons why experts think woman are twice as likely to experience depression as men. Although girls and boys have an equal risk for depression during childhood, the risk in women rises just after puberty, when their bodies start producing female hormones. The risk is also higher for some women during their menstrual period (premenstrual dysphoric disorder), after they give birth (postpartum depression) and while they are going through menopause—all of which involve hormonal shifts in a woman's body.

According to research out of Harvard Medical School in 2011, the hormone leptin has been linked with depression in women. This hormone is produced by human fat cells. In the study, women's blood levels of leptin were associated with symptoms of both anxiety and depression, and these associations were independent of the women's body weight or fat mass. The hormone leptin, which helps regulate body fat, has also been linked with depression in women (Box 1-8).

NEW FINDING

Box 1-8: Leptin linked with depression in women

According to research out of Harvard Medical School in 2011, the hormone leptin has been linked with depression in women. This hormone is produced by human fat cells. In the study, women's blood levels of leptin were associated with symptoms of both anxiety and depression and these associations were independent of the women's body weight or fat mass.

Box 1-9: Roots of depression—An intricate tapestry

The importance of the interaction of multiple factors leading to depression was highlighted by a study published in the November 2011 issue of *Human Brain Mapping*. For this study, French researchers scanned the brains of people who were carriers of a gene known to be implicated in depression as well as the brains of non-carriers. Carriers and non-carriers of the gene had different patterns of activation of their amygdala—a part of the brain known to be implicated in emotion—when they were shown pleasant or unpleasant images and asked to think about the links between the images they saw and themselves. Illustrating the interplay among environment, genes and the brain, stress experienced by the participants during the year prior to the test affected how the depression gene influenced the response of the amygdala.

Putting it all Together

For most people with depression, the cause is more complex than just unbalanced hormones or the wrong genes. Our genes, our bodies, our environment, our personality and our lifestyle all combine together in a way that can sometimes produce the condition (Box 1-9).

A relatively new field of science known as epigenetics is also helping to unravel the complicated relationship between our genes and our environment. Research in this field is demonstrating that our environment can directly impact how our genes function (Box 1-10).

In the next chapter we'll look at the different types of depression that exist, and the impact they can have on mood. ■

NEW FINDING

Box 1-10: Epigenetics helps clarify the nature/nurture debate over mental health

For decades researchers have argued about whether certain personality characteristics and illness are a result of our genes (nature) or environment (nature). Recently, it has become clear that, in fact, both genes and the environment interact constantly to make us who we are and produce illnesses such as depression.

Now, the new field of epigenetics demonstrates that the interaction is even more complex than we once thought. It turns out that certain environmental influences can actually make changes to our genes that affect how they function and that these changes can go on to be inherited by our offspring. Some of the most famous research in the field of epigenetics has come out of the lab of Dr. Michael Meaney at McGill University in Montreal. Dr. Meaney's research has shown that a lack of nurturing behavior among rat mothers with their pups actually produces changes in the NR3C1 gene. The affected pups live their lives in a physical state of stress even when their environments are not stressful.

To determine whether similar mechanisms are at play in humans, researchers out of the Douglas Hospital in Montreal have been testing the brains of suicide victims with a history of abuse in childhood, suicide victims with no such history and those who died of other causes. The investigators have found that similar changes to the very same NR3C1 gene occurred most frequently in suicide victims with a history of abuse, suggesting that their negative childhood experiences produced genetic changes that made them vulnerable to suicide later in life. And just as with the rats, the individuals with disrupted NR3C1 genes also lived in a state of constant physical stress.

Dr. Meaney and his team are continuing to look into the epigenetic underpinnings of mental health problems. They are following the children of mothers with severe depression. Frequently, depressed mothers are unable to provide their children with the nurturing they need. The investigators are testing levels of stress hormones and conducting brain imaging studies in these children to help determine whether their deprived environments have produced physiological changes that could set them up for a future of mental illness.

2 TYPES OF DEPRESSION

Depression isn't one condition that causes the exact same symptoms in everyone who has it. Several different forms of depression exist. The most common types of depression are major depression (also called clinical depression) and dysthymia (a form of milder chronic depression), but there are also other, less common forms. Each type of depression has its own unique symptoms and treatments.

Major Depressive Disorder

Major depressive disorder, or major depression, is the most common type of depression. It affects 15 million adults—5 to 8 percent of the U.S. population at any given time—according to the National Alliance on Mental Illness. About one in eight individuals will experience major depression sometime in their lives. People who have major depression aren't just sad for a few days. Their low mood lasts for at least two weeks and usually much longer and is significant enough to interfere with their thoughts, behavior and physical health. Usually, there are other symptoms in addition to low mood, including:

■ Appetite changes with weight loss or weight gain

■ Sleeping too little or too much

■ Trouble with concentration and/or memory

■ Unexplained aches and pains

■ Fatigue/lack of energy

■ Loss of interest in activities that were once pleasurable

■ Agitation, restlessness or irritability

■ Feelings of isolation or loneliness

■ Feelings of worthlessness, self-hate or guilt

■ Recurring thoughts of death or suicide

Although major depression can occur at any age, it's most common in people between the ages of 25 and 44. If you have one episode of major depression, you have a 50 percent chance of having another episode. The more episodes of major depression you have, the greater your odds of having another one.

Diseases That Can Complicate or Mimic Depression

A number of illnesses have symptoms that can mimic, cause, be a consequence of or complicate depression. That's why it's important to diagnose the underlying condition and to be alert for symptoms of depression.

Research finds that people who have depression along with a medical illness tend to have more symptoms of both conditions and more difficulty dealing with their illness. Treating the depression can also help improve the underlying medical condition.

Medical conditions that can cause depression include:

- Addison's disease
- AIDS
- Brain tumors
- Cancer
- Coronary artery disease
- Cushing's disease
- Diabetes
- Encephalitis
- Fibromyalgia
- Head trauma
- Heart disease
- Hypercalcemia (high levels of calcium in the blood)
- Hyperparathyroidism (overactive parathyroid glands)
- Hyperthyroidism (overactive thyroid glands)
- Hypothyroidism (underactive thyroid glands)
- Influenza (the flu)
- Kidney or liver failure
- Mononucleosis
- Multiple sclerosis
- Parkinson's disease
- Seizures
- Sleep apnea
- Stroke
- Systemic lupus erythematosus
- Tuberculosis
- Viral hepatitis
- Viral pneumonia
- Vitamin deficiencies (folate, B12, D)

A number of psychological conditions also can either stem from or contribute to depression. These include:

- Alcoholism and other substance abuse disorders
- Anxiety disorders—including post-traumatic stress disorder (PTSD), obsessive-compulsive disorder, social phobia and generalized anxiety disorder
- Eating disorders—including anorexia nervosa and bulimia nervosa
- Personality disorders—including borderline personality disorder

Dysthymia

When depression isn't severe enough to be called major depression, but it lingers for a long period of time, it is called dysthymia. The word comes from the Greek term meaning "bad state of mind." The official definition of dysthymia is having depressed mood nearly every day for at least two years, although it can last for much longer.

Just because dysthymia isn't as severe as major depression doesn't mean it isn't serious or disabling. If you have dysthymia, you'll experience many of the same symptoms as you would if you had major depression, such as a lack of energy, disturbed sleep, low self-esteem and an inability to concentrate. You'll also have some of the same detrimental effects on your life, including your performance at school and work and disturbances in your social relationships.

In addition, having dysthymia makes you more likely to develop major depression. More than half of people with dysthymia will also have at least one episode of major depression (which is called double depression when these conditions overlap).

Depression Related to Menstruation, Pregnancy and Birth

As mentioned earlier, hormones can play an important role in depression. That is why women can become vulnerable to the condition during periods of hormonal upset. One of these periods is during the days leading up to the commencement of the menstrual period. Hormonal changes can make women irritable, anxious or depressed. For up to 80 percent of American women, this is a normal part of life and nothing more than an inconvenience. But for 3 to 8 percent of women, these symptoms are severe enough during the premenstrual period to significantly interfere with everyday life but then diminish or disappear after menses have begun. These women are said to be suffering from premenstrual dysphoric disorder. This is a medical condition that frequently requires treatment. Sometimes women with premenstrual dysmorphic disorder do well simply by taking medication during the premenstrual period, when they are most vulnerable to depressed mood. Other women with the disorder may need to take medication all the time or try other treatments such as psychotherapy.

While news of pregnancy is usually a joyful event, for some mothers-to-be the hormone fluctuations of pregnancy and other factors such as the stress of an unplanned pregnancy can be overwhelming. About 13 percent of pregnant women and new mothers experience depression, according to the U.S. Department of Health and Human Services. Women from poorer socioeconomic backgrounds are at an even greater risk for depression during their pregnancy. It's especially important to get treated for depression while you're pregnant. Without treatment, depression can hurt not only you, but also your unborn baby. Pregnant women who are depressed are less likely to eat and sleep well. They tend to miss their prenatal visits and to use substances that are dangerous for the baby (such as alcohol, illegal drugs or tobacco). Babies born to depressed mothers are more likely to be premature and low birth weight. They may have delays in language development and increased behavioral problems. Depression during pregnancy is such a big concern that guidelines from the American College of Obstetricians and Gynecologists advise routinely screening women for depression both during and shortly after their pregnancy.

While experts recommend against taking medication during pregnancy whenever possible, they also acknowledge that the risks of letting depression go unchecked can be higher than the risk that medication for depression may have an undesirable effect on the developing baby. That's why it is important for pregnant women who are depressed to carefully discuss the pros and cons of various treatment options for depression with their physician.

Giving birth is an exciting time. You wait for nine long months until finally you're able to bring this amazing new person home. Being a new mother isn't easy, though, especially if this is your first time. It's very common for women to feel overwhelmed by all of their new responsibilities. You may feel sad or cry at the drop of a hat for the first few days after bringing home your new baby. These symptoms, termed the baby blues, are very common. They will go away on their own within a few days or a week as you settle into motherhood.

For about 10 percent of women, however, the baby blues are more severe and persist for more than a few days. This is called postpartum depression, and it brings with it overwhelming feelings of sadness, worthlessness and hopelessness. During pregnancy, levels of the female hormones estrogen and progesterone rise. Within 24 hours after delivery, levels of these hormones drop back to normal. Levels of other hormones, particularly thyroid hormones, also drop after childbirth. These quick plunges in hormone levels can trigger postpartum depression.

Having a new baby in the house can also lead to depression in other ways. New mothers may be exhausted from the many late-night feelings, overwhelmed by the responsibilities of caring for a new baby, frustrated at the change in their lifestyle (no longer being able to go to work or get out of the house) and upset by the changes in their body from pregnancy. These feelings can become even more intense if the mother isn't getting enough support from her spouse, friends and family. You're more likely to have postpartum depression if you've been depressed before, or if you are under a lot of stress (from marital or financial problems, for example).

New mothers aren't the only ones who suffer from postpartum depression. Fathers are also at greater risk for depression for several months and even years after their children are born. Fathers fall prey to depression for many of the same reasons mothers do: poor sleep, the stress of having a new baby in the house and increased demands on their time. Depression affects about 7 percent of new dads, and it can seriously impact their parenting skills.

As if caring for a new baby is stressful enough, having postpartum depression can make your new job even more difficult. Postpartum depression is increasingly recognized as a serious medical illness that poses risks to both mother and baby. It can interfere with the bonding between mother and baby, and a lack of attachment early on has been shown to contribute to numerous problems with the child's emotional and social development as well as with his or her learning ability later in childhood. That is why obstetricians are increasingly screening for postpartum depression.

Women shouldn't accept persistent low mood as an inevitable part of motherhood. Postpartum depression is treatable. Without treatment it can get worse and settle into long-term depression. Talk to your doctor about starting therapy or taking medications. If you are breastfeeding, your doctor will help you weigh the pros and cons of taking antidepressants. Research has suggested that skin-to-skin contact may alleviate postpartum blues (Box 2-1).

Postpartum depression is not the same as postpartum psychosis, a condition that affects about one out of every 1,000 women after they give birth. Women who have postpartum psychosis become very confused. They may hallucinate (see or hear things that aren't there) or have severe mood swings. Most importantly, they may try to hurt themselves or their new baby. This is a very serious condition. If you or someone you love has

NEW FINDING

Box 2-1: Skin-to-skin contact may alleviate postpartum depression

Depression in mothers in the weeks or months after childbirth, a condition known as postpartum *depression*, has been linked with several negative health outcomes for both mother and child. Finding ways to alleviate this form of depression is therefore a high priority. As trace amounts of certain antidepressants in breast milk may cause side effects in infants, approaches that minimize the use of medications during breastfeeding are desirable. Research published in the April 2012 issue of the *Journal of Obstetric, Gynecologic and Neonatal Nursing* suggests that simply encouraging skin-to-skin contact between mother and child can help alleviate the mental distress experienced by many women after they give birth.

For the study, 90 new mothers were randomly assigned to a group in which they were instructed to have at least five hours a day of skin-to-skin contact with their infants during the infants' first week of life and then at least two hours a day until the infant reached one month of age. The other group of women received no special instructions and experienced very little skin-to-skin contact with their infants.

The women who had the increased skin-to-skin contact had better scores on measurements of depression during their infants' first week of life and marginally better scores when their infants were one month old. They also had lower levels of the stress hormone cortisol in their saliva. The differences between the two groups of women disappeared after the enhanced skin-to-skin contact was discontinued. Nevertheless, it is important to keep in mind that although this study showed that skin-to-skin contact reduced depressive symptoms, it is not yet known whether this has a role in preventing serious depression in the form of postpartum depression.

any symptoms of postpartum psychosis (Box 2-2), call your doctor right away.

Psychotic Depression

People who are depressed may not feel like themselves. They often have exaggerated feelings of guilt or worthlessness and may be more sensitive to criticism or rejection. However, most people with major depression remain in touch with reality. Psychotic depression is a different story. In people who have this condition, depression is accompanied by strange hallucinations or delusions, which are often bizarre beliefs that have no basis in reality.

For example, a woman with the condition might be convinced that she is responsible for a dreadful but imaginary crime, that her internal organs are rotting inside her body or that the government has planted a chip inside her brain to monitor her thoughts. She may hear voices that confirm these beliefs. Unlike with other psychotic conditions such as schizophrenia, people who have psychotic depression often recognize that their thoughts are distorted and may try to hide those thoughts from other people.

Experts say psychotic depression is more common than most people think, affecting up to 25 percent of people with severe, hospital-level

BOX 2-2: "BABY BLUES," POSTPARTUM DEPRESSION OR POSTPARTUM PSYCHOSIS: HOW TO TELL THE DIFFERENCE

CONDITION	WHEN IT OCCURS	HOW LONG IT LASTS	SYMPTOMS	
"Baby blues"	Three to five days after the baby is born	Less than two weeks after delivery	■ Sadness ■ Crying for no reason ■ Irritability ■ Anxiety	■ Fatigue ■ Insomnia ■ Mood changes
Postpartum depression	One to three weeks after delivery	May last several months to a year, especially when untreated	■ Depressed mood ■ Loss of interest in activities you once enjoyed ■ Appetite changes	■ Sleep problems ■ Lack of energy ■ Feelings of worthlessness or guilt ■ Difficulty concentrating
Postpartum psychosis	During the first three weeks after childbirth	Psychosis may continue without treatment	■ Extreme confusion ■ Feeling detached from your baby and other people ■ Dramatically changing moods	■ Bizarre behavior ■ Agitation ■ Hallucinations ■ Thoughts of hurting yourself and/or the baby

depression. Yet relatively little research has been done on this condition and no medication is specifically approved for treating it. Usually, treatment involves combining antidepressant and antipsychotic medications. Sometimes additional treatment is needed, such electroconvulsive therapy (see Chapter 5).

Bipolar Disorder (Manic Depressive Illness)

Most people live their lives on a pretty even keel. Day-to-day their temperament remains similar, although they may experience periods of happiness and sadness in response to life events. For people with bipolar disorder, however, life is often a rollercoaster ride. Their moods may shift radically from week to week.

During the high points, people with bipolar disorder may be almost euphorically happy and full of energy, sleep little or not at all for days on end, engage in reckless behavior, have intense flashes of irritability and have grandiose beliefs about themselves. They may also have racing, disorganized thoughts and speak almost too quickly to be understood. This is known as a manic episode. As with severe depression, sometimes people in a manic stage of bipolar disorder hallucinate or have delusions.

Manic episodes, or more subtle episodes that have similar features but are less intense (called hypomanic episodes), typically last from four or five days to a few weeks. Unfortunately, when they subside, the person often plunges into the deepest depths of a depressive episode.

During "pure" episodes of depression, the symptoms of bipolar disorder are hard to distinguish from the symptoms of major depression. The person will often feel sad, tired, withdrawn and will have trouble concentrating, sleeping and eating. He or she may experience thoughts of worthlessness, guilt, death or suicide. Although mania is a defining feature of bipolar disorder, most individuals with bipolar disorder experience depression far more frequently and for much longer periods of time than they experience mania.

Although manic and depressive episodes usually alternate with one another, doctors now recognize that in some people, bipolar disorder appears as a mixture of the two states: mania and depression. During these mixed episodes, a person can experience the elements of mania (such as high energy, physical restlessness and impulsivity) at the same time as the symptoms of depression (such as sadness, guilt or suicidal urges). Not only are mixed states more common than was once thought, they may be particularly dangerous because the person's energy level is high enough for them to act on their negative thoughts.

Understandably, swinging between such extremes in mood and behavior can severely disrupt a person's life, work and relationships. During the manic or mixed episodes, the almost frantic energy level and impulsive, risky behaviors can overwhelm friends, family members and co-workers, sometimes ending promising careers and marriages. During the depressive episodes, the person may withdraw completely and spend days on end in bed. It's common for people with bipolar disorder to abuse alcohol or drugs, perform poorly in school or work and have relationship conflicts. Treatment with mood stabilizing medication and therapy can help people with bipolar disorder lead a more balanced life by regulating their moods and improving their relationships.

Research is finding that some people with major depression may actually have a "hidden" form of bipolar disorder. In a 2010 study that involved more than 9,200 people, nearly 40 percent of the people who had a history of major depressive disorder described periods of hypomania that fall just under the radar for an official diagnosis of bipolar disorder, a condition called subthreshold hypomania. The authors say the criteria for bipolar disorder should be broadened, because some patients with subthreshold hypomania might also benefit from taking a mood stabilizing medication after they are treated with antidepressants.

Seasonal Affective Disorder (SAD)

Winter can be a depressing time, especially if you live in a cold northern climate. It's easy to feel sad when the long, dark days and frigid temperatures keep you cooped up inside. Just about everyone has had the "winter blues" at one time or another. Yet in some people, the sadness that creeps in during the winter months goes far beyond the blues. Every winter, like clockwork, they feel moody, anxious and tired and they lose interest in activities they once loved. They retreat into their winter hibernation and don't become their old selves again until the first buds of spring appear.

Depression that occurs exclusively with the change of seasons is called seasonal affective disorder, or SAD. Researchers believe that the lack of sunlight in the winter disrupts the body's natural internal clock (circadian rhythm), which determines when you sleep and when you are awake. For some people, lower vitamin D levels that are more likely to occur in the northern winters may also contribute to the risk for depressive symptoms.

Usually SAD sets in during the winter months and improves by spring, but some people experience mood swings during the summer months. Summer-onset SAD may be due to malaise brought on by rising heat and humidity. Whereas people with winter-onset SAD experience a drop in energy, those with summer-onset SAD tend to be more irritable and anxious. The symptoms of depression are generally mild in people with SAD, but they keep returning, year after year. Most likely, the number of people who have "pure" SAD is small in comparison with the number of people with major depression whose mood is partly influenced by the change in seasons.

Substance-Induced Depression

As mentioned earlier, use of certain medications and illicit drugs can lead to depression. When this happens, a person is said to have substance-induced depression. This type of depression is considered separate from other types of depression because both the cause and treatment are typically different from naturally occurring depression. In particular, whenever possible the offending drug, if prescribed, is discontinued or the dose is reduced. If the drug causing the depression is being abused, the person will likely require some form of addiction treatment (drug rehab) in order to recover completely.

Although substance-induced depression is a separate category of depression, some individuals truly have a dual diagnosis. They have depression as well as a substance use disorder. It is sometimes difficult to know for sure which came first but both conditions hinder recovery from the other and both require treatment. Fortunately, dual diagnosis treatment programs exist where expertise exists for treating both mood disorders and substance use concurrently.

Atypical and Melancholic Depression

Depression isn't a one-size-fits-all diagnosis. That means not everyone will experience its symptoms in exactly the same way. Some researchers over the years have made a distinction between people with two different types of depression symptoms. There are depressed people who:

■ Lose appetite and weight

■ Sleep poorly

■ Have strong feelings of guilt

■ Don't respond at all to pleasurable events when they are depressed

There are also depressed people who:

■ Gain weight and crave carbohydrates (such as cereals, bread, pasta and sweets)

■ Oversleep

■ Have heavy sensations in their limbs (leaden paralysis)

■ Become less depressed, although transiently, when exposed to pleasurable events (mood reactivity)

■ Have enhanced reactions to criticism or rejection (rejection sensitivity)

The former kind of depression is referred to as melancholic depression, while the latter form of depression is called atypical depression.

Some research has suggested that certain medications (such as the monoamine oxidase inhibitors) may be more effective than others (such as the tricyclic antidepressants) for atypical depression. However, it is not clear whether melancholic and atypical depression are truly different forms of major depressive disorder with different causes and treatments, or whether they are simply different ways that depression can manifest itself among the millions of people who suffer from it.

Researchers are describing and studying other potential subtypes of depression, as well. These subtypes include:

■ Anxious depression

■ Depression with anger attacks

■ Early-onset (child/adolescent) depression

As with atypical and melancholic depression, it is unclear whether these newer subtypes are truly different forms of depression.

Just as the signs and symptoms of depression can differ from one person to another, the impact of depression can also differ across people. In the next chapter, we'll look at the unique ways in which depression affects men, women, children, older adults and different cultural groups. ■

3 HOW DEPRESSION AFFECTS DIFFERENT PEOPLE

Depression unquestionably affects people's lives in many different ways, but the impact is not the same for everyone. Different cultures, genders and ages experience depression in unique ways. In this chapter, we'll look at the different effects of depression on women, men, children and older adults.

Who Does Depression Affect?

Depression affects nearly one in 10, or 9 percent of American adults, including 4 percent who have major depression, according to the Centers for Disease Control and Prevention (CDC). Rates of depression are highest among young adults (ages 18 to 24) and middle-aged people (ages 45 to 64). Women are more likely to experience depression than men, and people with little education face a greater incidence of depression than those who have completed at least some college. African-Americans are the ethnic group most likely to have depression, followed by Hispanics and Caucasians.

People who live in the South face the greatest risk for depression. Alabama, Arkansas, Louisiana, Mississippi, Oklahoma, Tennessee and West Virginia have the highest rates. North Dakota, Michigan, Alaska, Colorado, Minnesota, Iowa and Connecticut are among the states with the lowest rates of depression.

Impact of Depression

When you're down day after day, just getting out of bed in the morning seems like a chore. As you move wearily through your day, your depression has an impact on just about every aspect of your life. It could even threaten your life.

Work

Depression drains energy and saps concentration. It's no wonder, then, that people who are depressed are less productive at their jobs. They are also absent more often from work. Depression is the leading cause of disability among Americans ages 15 to 44, according to the National Institute of Mental Health. Workers who are depressed are about twice as likely as their colleagues to use short-term disability leave, even if they are receiving treatment. Studies find that time lost from depression costs employers more than $40 billion a year. Even when compared with other important medical conditions including heart disease, arthritis, cancer and accidents, depression is a leading cause of work disability throughout the world.

Relationships

Depression has a ripple effect in families. When one member is depressed, the repercussions eventually reach everyone in the household. Say, for example, a father is depressed. He withdraws from his wife and children. He eats and sleeps too much, neglecting his appearance and his health. He could have temper outbursts. His wife might be sympathetic and pick up the slack at first, but eventually she becomes angry and resentful. His children will ask him to play with them several times before they finally give up and feel neglected. The rift that depression creates will continue to grow unless the husband gets treated. Depression affects not only marriages, but also relationships with friends, co-workers and other family members.

Social stigma

No matter how far the field of psychology has progressed, depression and other mental health conditions still carry a social stigma. The embarrassment associated with having depression, along with difficulties in finding access to depression therapy, may be why an estimated 50 percent of Americans with depression don't seek the treatment they need.

Suicide

When depression is not treated, the emotional anguish can become unbearable. Some people who are depressed become so overwhelmed by a profound sense of worthlessness, guilt or emptiness that they would rather die than endure another day. More than 90 percent of people who commit suicide have clinical depression or another mental illness. Those who are depressed become even more likely to commit suicide if they experience a traumatic life event, such as the death of a loved one or the breakup of a relationship. If you or a loved one has any thoughts about suicide, it's crucial to get help right away. (See Chapter 6 for the warning signs of suicidal tendencies and how to find support).

Cultural Differences

Cultural differences can have a profound impact on how people experience and interpret depression. In Asia, for example, people are more likely to experience depression through physical symptoms such as aches and pains, weakness and fatigue or dizziness. In the Middle East, people describe their depression as a kind of heartbreak. In some cultures, depression is not as widely discussed or studied. Perhaps this is why in Japan women with depression often complain of shoulder pain, which they refer to as "futeishuso," meaning "nonspecific complaint."

A person's culture can also determine his or her response to depression. Although African Americans generally experience major depression more often than Caucasians, they are less likely to seek help when they are depressed. African Americans are only about half as likely as Caucasians and Puerto Ricans to get the kind of therapy recommended by the American Psychiatric Association. The disparity may be due, in part, to a lack of insurance coverage, as well as to other factors.

Every depressed individual is unique, defying simple stereotypes. Still, people from diverse cultural backgrounds can often benefit from the care of a mental health professional who appreciates cultural differences and who understands how cultural background influences a person's ability to cope with, and get treated for depression.

Depression in Women

There is a real gender gap when it comes to depression. Women face double the risk of the condition compared to men, particularly after they give birth or as they are entering into the hormonal changes that precede menopause. Women are more vulnerable to depression than men in part due to hormonal differences and in part due to the way women deal emotionally with stressful life events (such as a divorce or the loss of a loved one). Depression often coexists with other health and mental conditions that have a higher prevalence in women, such as eating disorders, anxiety disorders and multiple sclerosis.

The symptoms of depression are also different in women than they are in men. Women are more likely to experience anxiety and physical symptoms. They also tend to overeat and gain more weight. There is a close relationship between obesity and depression, particularly in women. Obese women are nearly four times more likely to be depressed than women who are of normal weight. The same association doesn't seem to be true for obese men. It may be that women feel more of a societal pressure to be thin than do men, and doctors may need to screen for depression more often in obese women.

Unfortunately, depression can take a big toll on women. Depression is the number one cause of disability in women. Though more men actually take their own lives, women attempt suicide about twice as often. Depression has been linked with a higher risk of coronary heart disease and of sudden cardiac death in women. Yet despite these many risks, fewer than half of women with clinical depression ever seek treatment.

Depression in Men

Although women face double the risk, depression isn't solely a women's condition. More than 6 million men contend with depression every year. How that depression manifests in men is different than in women, however. While women tend to turn their emotions inward and feel worthless and guilty, men tend to reflect their emotions outward, sometimes becoming angry and even aggressive.

Because men are traditionally perceived as the "stronger," more "stoic" gender, they are more likely to gloss over depression symptoms such as a lack of interest in life, fatigue and low self-esteem. They might fear that revealing their condition will make them look "weak" or "overly emotional" to their family, friends and colleagues.

Instead of acknowledging their depression and seeking professional help, often men turn to alcohol or drugs for relief. Without treatment, their depression can become a crushing weight. Eventually it can send men into a dangerous emotional spiral that ends in violence against themselves or others.

Depression in the Elderly

Age undoubtedly brings wisdom, but it doesn't always bring contentment. Growing older can introduce many new stresses into a person's life, such as getting accustomed to retirement, moving to a new home, or dealing with the idea that children have less time for them because they are wrapped up with their own growing families and careers. There may be financial concerns after retirement, especially if investments have lost value and medical bills are piling up. There may be physical limitations from diseases that are more common with advancing age, such as arthritis, Parkinson's disease or stroke. There can be grief and sadness that comes with the loss of friends, family members, or a spouse. Finally, neurological and other health changes that occur with age can make people more vulnerable to depression and vice versa. Stroke, which occurs more commonly with advancing age, can produce neurological changes that make one vulnerable to depression. Cognitive decline and dementia are intimately intertwined in older people. In fact, the symptoms of each can be difficult to tease apart, and one frequently worsens the other. On the flip side of the coin, depression experienced in mid-life and late-life has been linked with an increased risk of developing dementia in older age (Box 3-1).

For all of these reasons, depression affects more than 6.5 million of those aged 65 and older, according to the National Alliance on Mental Illness. That number rises dramatically among elderly people who are hospitalized—illustrating the effect significant illness can have on mental health.

Although many depression triggers occur with age, the idea that low mood is a normal part of aging is a misperception that leads to many missed opportunities for diagnosis and effective treatment.

The implications of depression on seniors are especially profound because depression can quicken cognitive decline and exacerbate illness. It also can increase the risk for suicide among the elderly. Older white men face the highest suicide rate of any group in the U.S. Sadly, many older adults reach out for help in the days or weeks before they attempt suicide but don't seem to find it.

Depression in Children

All children get sad from time to time. Often they seem to respond dramatically to the littlest things, like losing a toy or not getting their favorite dessert. Yet for some children, low mood is an everyday occurrence. About 5 percent of children and adolescents are depressed at any given time, according to the American Academy of Child & Adolescent Psychiatry.

Up to around age 10, depression occurs about equally in boys and girls. During adolescence, though, the condition becomes increasingly prevalent in girls, especially after the hormonal changes that occur around the time of a girl's first menstrual period.

Box 3-2: Depression and social relationships in childhood are a two-way street

In a 2012 study published in the journal *Child Development*, children who were depressed in Grade 4 were found to be at increased risk of being victimized by peers the following year, and this in turn predicted the likelihood that they would have difficulty being accepted by peers in Grade 6. These findings call into question the assumption that there is a one-way association between lack of peer acceptance and depression. In fact, either one can lead to the other. This is why it is important to address both social problems and signs of depression in children as early as possible. Early intervention can help prevent the problem from compounding over time.

Just as in adults, depression in children stems from a combination of factors:

■ Genetics: Children of depressed parents are more likely to become depressed themselves.

■ Environment: Depression is more common in children with unstable or abusive families and in those who are under other forms of stress.

■ Personal history: Kids who have behavioral or anxiety disorders are more likely to be depressed.

■ Brain chemistry: Neurotransmitter imbalances can affect mood in children, just as they do in adults.

Children—especially young children—may have more trouble articulating that they are upset. Their symptoms may not fit the typical pattern of adult depression. For example, a child might seem bored or angry rather than sad. Depressed kids also tend to complain of physical ailments like stomachaches or headaches because they aren't able to accurately express their emotions.

Some children's expression of depression can be so different from that of adults that experts have proposed a new type of depression that more closely fits what is sometimes seen in children. This new subtype is known as disruptive mood regulation disorder and is characterized by a mood that is persistently angry or irritable combined with regular outbursts of temper. This condition is believed to appear for the first time among children aged 6 to 18.

In children and adolescents, problems with depression frequently go hand-in hand with problems with social relationships (Box 3-2).

You'll learn more about the symptoms of depression in children and adults in the next chapter. ■

4 DIAGNOSING DEPRESSION

You're sad. You're listless. You no longer have any interest in going out with friends. You're tired, and have lost weight without trying. Are you just in a funk or are you really depressed? If you've been feeling this way for at least two weeks, it could be depression.

The only way to know for sure is to see your doctor or a mental health professional and get diagnosed (Boxes 4-1 and 4-2).

Once your doctor determines that you are depressed and figures out what kind of depression you have, you can get the right treatment.

BOX 4-1

Specialists who treat depression

■ **PSYCHIATRIST:** These physicians (MDs) specialize in the prevention, treatment and diagnosis of mental disorders. Psychiatrists are able to prescribe medications for depression. They may also treat patients with talk therapy or refer patients to psychologists, social workers or other mental health professionals for talk therapy. They must be licensed to practice in the state in which they work. Psychiatrists may also be certified by the American Board of Psychiatry and Neurology.

■ **PSYCHOLOGIST:** These specialists typically hold a doctorate degree (PhD, PsyD, or EdD) or master's degree in psychology. Psychologists can diagnose depression using various tests, and they can treat the condition with talk therapy. In most states, they cannot prescribe drugs but often refer patients who need medication to psychiatrists, primary care doctors or nurse practitioners. Psychologists must be licensed by their state and certified by the American Board of Professional Psychology.

■ **THERAPIST:** "Therapist" is a broad and non-specific term for professionals who provide support to families, groups or individuals. Therapists may have some form of certification and licensure. Many, but not all therapists are social workers, psychologists or psychiatrists. However, there are therapists (such as certain mental health or addiction counselors) who do not have a master's, doctorate or MD degree but have completed shorter, specialized training programs. If you choose to see a therapist, it's a good idea to ask about their training and experience in treating depression.

■ **PSYCHIATRIC NURSE:** Psychiatric nurses are specialized nurses who treat people with depression and other mental health issues. They hold a degree in nursing, are licensed as registered nurses (RN), and have additional training in psychiatry. In some states, psychiatric nurses can prescribe medications, but usually only under a doctor's supervision.

■ **SOCIAL WORKER:** Social workers hold a master's degree in social work and are trained in psychotherapy. Most states require them to be licensed or certified. Clinical social workers often work for hospitals or social services agencies. They help ensure that patients get access to the care they need. Like psychologists, social workers work closely with a psychiatrist, primary care doctor or nurse practitioner if patients need medications along with talk therapy to treat their depression

BOX 4-2

Choosing the right mental health professional

Many primary care doctors, nurse practitioners and doctors in other fields, such as pediatrics, gynecology or neurology, are trained to recognize and potentially treat depression. But more severe depression that does not respond to usual treatments or that is complicated by medical illness may require a referral to a mental health professional who is trained in the evaluation and treatment of depression.

If you are interested in psychotherapy instead of or in addition to medication, you will need to work with a mental health professional.

Here are some tips for finding the psychiatrist, psychologist or other mental health professional who best fits your needs:

Referrals: Ask your primary care physician for a referral. You may also wish to contact your insurance company for information about local providers with expertise in depression. The American Psychological Association or American Psychiatric Association has listings of psychologists and psychiatrists in your area. Many hospitals and health centers have departments of psychiatry or divisions of mental health that can offer information on local resources. Increasingly, hospitals have their own specialized depression treatment and research centers.

Health insurance: When you make your appointment, ask whether the specialist accepts your health insurance.

Area of expertise: Ask about the mental health professional's areas of expertise (including types of mental health problems treated and kinds of treatment offered), professional degrees held and number of years in practice.

Personality and style: When you meet with the mental health professional for the first time, make sure you are comfortable with his or her personality and style.

Treatment recommendation: After you have your first session, ask what treatment or range of treatments your clinician recommends and how long treatment will take. It's also a good idea to ask how long before you should expect to start feeling better once treatment has begun.

Be candid with your mental health professional.

If you are skeptical of or surprised by the diagnosis, tell your mental health professional.

If the treatment recommended (such as antidepressants or talk therapy) differs from the treatment you expected or prefer, discuss this. Perhaps the treatment you prefer would be an equally valid starting point.

If you anticipate obstacles to sticking with treatment (such as side effects or challenges with transportation or insurance coverage), talk with your clinician to find a treatment that will work for you and make a plan that will help you overcome obstacles along the way.

Depression will not always respond to the first series of treatments, despite your best efforts and the best efforts of your mental health professional. Occasionally you may reach an impasse where depression persists, and you and your clinician may feel like you are at a loss for new ideas. When this happens, consider getting a "consultation" with another mental health professional. A fresh perspective can help shed light on factors (such as psychotic symptoms or hypothyroidism) that may be contributing to your depression, or enable you to consider potentially effective treatments that you haven't yet tried.

Symptoms of Depression

Not everyone experiences depression in the same way. While some people may feel down, others may appear angry. Some people may gorge themselves when they're feeling sad. Others can't eat anything. Depression can manifest as physical symptoms such as a headache or stomachache, or as emotional symptoms like crying and withdrawing from friends and family.

Depending on an individual's personality type, it can sometimes be hard to spot depression. When a person is always outgoing and upbeat, his or her friends and family may not recognize depression when it occurs. That's why it's important to be vigilant for the signs of depression—whether in yourself, a friend or a family member.

Because different genders and age groups experience depression in different ways, we have included a list of typical symptoms, as well as some of the less common symptoms certain groups of people might experience.

The most typical symptoms of depression include:
- Feeling sad, down or blue most of the time
- Loss of interest in activities and hobbies you once enjoyed
- Difficulty concentrating, paying attention and remembering
- Disrupted sleep (difficulty getting to sleep or staying asleep, or sleeping too much)
- Change in eating habits (overeating or losing your appetite)
- Fatigue and loss of energy
- Feelings of guilt or worthlessness
- Feelings of helplessness or hopelessness
- Increased alcohol and drug use
- Irritability
- Low self-esteem
- Neglecting your personal care (such as personal hygiene)
- Physical symptoms that don't respond to treatment (headaches, stomachaches, chronic pain)
- Reduced sex drive
- Thoughts of death or suicide

Less common symptoms of depression:
- Being highly sensitive to rejection or criticism, while perking up briefly with positive events

- Eating too much (often craving foods that are rich in carbohydrates such as ice cream, chocolate, bread, cereal and pasta)
- Feeling weighed down or heavy
- Sleeping too much

Symptoms of depression in the elderly:

- Confusion
- Difficulty sleeping
- Hallucinations or delusions (in depression with psychotic features)
- Irritability
- Loss of appetite and weight loss
- Memory problems
- Vague physical complaints
- Withdrawal from society

Symptoms of depression in children:

- Aches and pains (stomachache, headache) that don't respond to treatment
- Anger, irritability
- Changes in appetite
- Crying or yelling outbursts
- Disrupted sleep
- Persistent sadness
- Thoughts of death
- Withdrawal from friends and family

Are You Depressed?

Take the simple test in Box 4-3 to find out whether you might be depressed.

If you check off at least five items on this list and you've been experiencing these symptoms for at least two weeks, it's time to see your primary care doctor or a mental health specialist (psychiatrist or psychologist) for an evaluation.

The doctor will start by asking about your symptoms and for how long you've had them. You'll also discuss your medical history and any personal or family history of depression.

Screening questionnaires

Your doctor may also use screening questionnaires to supplement the clinical interview. Guidelines from the American Psychiatric Association recommend that people with major depressive disorder complete a rating scale—either administered by their doctor or that they take themselves—to assess the type, frequency and severity of their symptoms. Using a rating scale to evaluate symptoms can help the mental health professional tailor the treatment plan specifically to you. Rating scales may include any of the following:

Patient Health Questionnaire (PHQ 9)

This self-test contains nine items that assess depression symptoms. It can help diagnose depression and then evaluate the severity to help your doctor select the most appropriate treatment and monitor your progress while you are being treated.

Quick Inventory for Depressive Symptomatology

Self-Report (QIDS SR) is a 16-item self-test that is translated into multiple languages (www.ids-qids.org). It is used to assess a broad range of depression symptoms, and it can be used to track treatment response.

Beck Depression Inventory (BDI)

This classic depression self-test contains 21 questions that assess the intensity of depression. Each item includes a list of four statements that refer to one symptom of depression. Statements are listed by increasing severity.

Center for Epidemiologic Studies-Depression Scale (CES-D)

The CES-D has been around since the 1970s, and it remains one of the most widely used methods for assessing the symptoms of depression. On this test, you will be asked to check off which of 20 statements you have felt in the past one to seven days. Examples of statements on the scale include, "I felt that everything I did was an effort," or "I felt that people dislike me."

Hamilton Rating Scale for Depression (HRSD), also known as the Hamilton Depression Rating Scale (HDRS) or HAM-D

A psychologist or psychiatrist administers this 21-question scale to assess the severity of depression in people who have already been diagnosed. Each item ranks the severity of symptoms such as depressed mood, feelings of guilt and difficulty in work and activities.

Zung Self-Rating Depression Scale

The Zung scale is a 20-question assessment. The user checks off how often he or she has experienced certain symptoms, such as feeling downhearted, having crying spells or having trouble sleeping (Box 4-4 on the next page).

BOX 4-4: ZUNG SELF-RATING DEPRESSION SCALE

Name _____ Age _____ Sex _____ Date _____

	None or little of the time	Some of the time	Good part of the time	Most of the time
1. I feel down-hearted and blue.				
2. Morning is when I feel the best.				
3. I have crying spells or feel like it.				
4. I have trouble sleeping at night.				
5. I eat as much as I used to.				
6. I still enjoy sex.				
7. I notice that I am losing weight.				
8. I have trouble with constipation.				
9. My heart beats faster than usual.				
10. I get tired for no reason.				
11. My mind is as clear as it used to be.				
12. I find it easy to do the things I used to.				
13. I am restless and can't keep still.				
14. I feel hopeful about the future.				
15. I am more irritable than usual.				
16. I find it easy to make decisions.				
17. I feel that I am useful and needed.				
18. My life is pretty full.				
19. I feel that others would be better off if I were dead.				
20. I still enjoy the things I used to do.				

SDS Raw Score _____

Key for scoring the Self-Rating Depression Scale (SDS)

SDS item number	None or little of the time	Some of the time	Good part of the time	Most of the time	SDS item number	None or little of the time	Some of the time	Good part of the time	Most of the time
1.	1	2	3	4	11.	4	3	2	1
2.	4	3	2	1	12.	4	3	2	1
3.	1	2	3	4	13.	1	2	3	4
4.	1	2	3	4	14.	4	3	2	1
5.	4	3	2	1	15.	1	2	3	4
6.	4	3	2	1	16.	4	3	2	1
7.	1	2	3	4	17.	4	3	2	1
8.	1	2	3	4	18.	4	3	2	1
9.	1	2	3	4	19.	1	2	3	4
10.	1	2	3	4	20.	4	3	2	1

SDS index and equivalent clinical global impressions:

Below 50.............Within normal range
50-59 ....Minimal to mild depression
60-69 ....Moderate to marked depression
70 and over........Severe to extreme depression

Rating scales cannot diagnose depression on their own, which is why it is so important to have a full clinical evaluation. However, rating scales are helpful for assessing how severe your depression is at any given point and then evaluating how well you are responding to your treatment, whether it involves medications, psychotherapy, meditation, exercise or watchful waiting.

Physical exam and diagnostic tests

In addition to having a detailed interview, you may need a physical examination and diagnostic tests to rule out illnesses that cause symptoms of depression, such as a thyroid problem, stroke, central nervous system tumor, head injury or multiple sclerosis. People with typical depression usually do not need to have a detailed physical work-up, but those with complex medical problems or whose symptoms do not neatly fit the diagnosis of depression (for example, they have fatigue and weight loss without sadness or loss of interest) should have a physical exam

Diagnostic tests may include:

Blood tests

The following blood tests can be done to check for medical conditions that can cause depression symptoms:

- Levels of hormones, such as thyroid hormone
- Calcium levels
- Blood sugar (glucose) levels
- Liver and kidney function tests
- Complete blood count (CBC)
- Levels of vitamins such as B12, folate and vitamin D
- Test for inflammatory problems, such as erythrocyte sedimentation rate (ESR)

Although blood tests can check for medical conditions, they currently can't diagnose depression. But that may change in the future. Researchers are studying genetic variations that may eventually help identify depression.

For instance, Dutch researchers have identified a set of seven genes in the blood, which they have used to differentiate patients with major depression from healthy individuals. Newer research continues to identify potential blood markers for depression (Box 4-5).

While none of these blood tests are ready for widespread use, their successful development during the coming years could help revolutionize both the diagnosis and management of depression.

Imaging tests

Imaging tests such as an MRI or computed tomography (CT) scan of the brain may be ordered to rule out tumors, bleeding or neurological disorders such as multiple sclerosis. Imaging tests may also include a carotid ultrasound to check for blocked arteries in the neck that supply blood to the brain.

Electrophysiological tests

Certain forms of tests of electrical waves in the brain or heart are sometimes used to evaluate depression:

- Electroencephalogram (EEG) is used to rule out a seizure disorder (epilepsy).
- Electrocardiogram (ECG) is used to diagnose heart problems.

Neuropsychological testing

Neuropsychological testing may help to diagnose cognitive and memory complaints.

Sleep study

A polysomnography, or sleep study, may help uncover reasons for interrupted sleep or unusual daytime drowsiness, such as obstructive sleep apnea, restless legs or narcolepsy. These conditions may contribute to or mimic the symptoms of depression.

Medication or drug testing

Tests may be ordered to check blood levels of certain medications, or to look for drugs and other substances that may cause or worsen depression symptoms.

Testing for infections

Your doctor may order tests to check for certain types of infections that can affect brain function and behavior, such as HIV, syphilis or Lyme disease.

Diagnosing Depression in Children and Adolescents

Too often, the signs of depression in its youngest sufferers are overlooked. Children and adolescents who don't get properly diagnosed can't get the treatment they need. Adolescents who aren't treated for depression tend to do poorly in school and in social relationships. They complain more often of physical illness, and they are more likely to abuse drugs, become pregnant or commit suicide. For these reasons, the U.S. Preventive Services Task Force recommends that primary care physicians routinely screen all of their teenage patients for major depression.

Although the Task Force says there isn't enough evidence currently to recommend the same screening for children under age 12, parents of young children should be on the lookout for the symptoms of depression listed above and should contact their child's pediatrician if they are seeing these symptoms on a regular basis.

Diagnosing depression in children starts with a detailed medical, developmental and mental health history. The doctor will ask when the child's symptoms started, how long they have lasted, how often they occur and how intense they are. The doctor might also request tests to rule out medical conditions with symptoms similar to those of depression.

In young children (ages 6 to 12), parents may be asked to fill out a 35-item Pediatric Symptom Checklist to assess how well their child is functioning psychologically and socially. Older children may be asked to fill out some of the same questionnaires used to diagnose depression in adults, such as the Beck Depression Inventory.

Part of the evaluation may include an interview with a child psychologist or psychiatrist. With very young children, this interview can involve having the child play, or the psychiatrist might observe as the child and parents interact. School-aged children may be asked questions directly. The doctor might also interview an adolescent or teen.

Now you've learned the various ways in which doctors diagnose depression and how to spot the signs in yourself or a loved one. In the next chapter, you'll see the treatments that can change the lives of people with depression. ◼

5 TREATMENTS FOR DEPRESSION

Getting diagnosed with depression is an important first step. The second step is to get treatment. It is very important that you take this second step. Depression is unlikely to go away if you ignore it—even if it's mild to start. Mild depression that isn't treated is likely to become major depression over time. Untreated depression often leads to growing problems at home and work. It may contribute to alcohol or drug use, and it can take a major toll on your physical health.

According to the National Institute for Mental Health, just over half of adult Americans suffering from depression receive what is considered to be "minimally adequate treatment" in any given 12-month period. That means nearly half of depressed people in the U.S. are not receiving the care they need, even though multiple effective therapies are available. Minority groups are particularly unlikely to receive the treatment they need. Don't let yourself become a victim of that statistic. If you or someone you love is depressed, get help.

There are many options for treating depression, from antidepressants to psychotherapy (talk therapy). Yet there isn't a single "one-size-fits-all" treatment. To find the treatment that will work best for your type and severity of depression, you'll need to work closely with your doctor.

Medication

Antidepressant medications are thought to improve mood by adjusting levels of the brain chemicals (neurotransmitters) that contribute to feelings of depression. Although these drugs can be very effective at combating depression, they can have side effects. Antidepressants can also interact with other drugs you are taking. It is very important that you check with your doctor and pharmacist to make sure that the antidepressant you are taking doesn't interact with any of your other medications (including over-the-counter drugs) or any vitamins or supplements you might be taking.

Antidepressants

Antidepressants are usually the first drugs prescribed for depression. Because the different types of antidepressant drugs have similar effectiveness, which medication your doctor prescribes will largely depend on the side effects and how well you tolerate the drug. Here is a rundown of the different antidepressant medications available, their benefits and potential side effects (Box 5-1):

BOX 5-1: ANTIDEPRESSANT MEDICATIONS

ANTIDEPRESSANT CLASS	MEDICATIONS IN THIS CLASS	SIDE EFFECTS		
Selective serotonin reuptake inhibitors (SSRIs)	• Citalopram (Celexa) • Escitalopram (Lexapro) • Fluoxetine (Prozac) • Fluvoxamine (Luvox) • Paroxetine (Paxil) • Sertraline (Zoloft) • Vilazodone (Viibryd)	• Agitation • Difficulty sleeping • Diarrhea • Drowsiness • Dry mouth • Headache • Increased sweating	• Interactions with other drugs • Nausea • Nervousness • Rash • Sexual problems	**Symptoms when you stop the drug abruptly:** • Nausea • Dizziness • Muscle pain • Headache
Serotonin-norepinephrine reuptake inhibitors (SNRIs)	• Duloxetine (Cymbalta) • Venlafaxine (Effexor) • Desvenlafaxine (Pristiq)	• Agitation or anxiety • Blurred or double vision • Constipation • Dizziness • Drowsiness • Dry mouth	• Elevated blood pressure • Insomnia • Nausea and vomiting • Sexual problems	**Symptoms when you stop the drug abruptly:** • Nausea • Dizziness • Muscle pain • Headache
Others	• Mirtazapine (Remeron)	• Constipation • Dizziness	• Drowsiness • Dry mouth	• Increased appetite • Weight gain
Norepinephrine-dopamine reuptake inhibitor	• Bupropion (Wellbutrin)	• Appetite loss • Dizziness • Dry mouth • Fast heartbeat • Frequent urination	• Headache • Muscle pain • Nausea and vomiting • Nervousness, agitation, anxiety	• Rash • Seizures • Sweating • Trouble sleeping • Weight loss
Reuptake inhibitors and receptor blockers	• Nefazodone (Serzone) • Trazodone (Desyrel)	• Constipation • Dizziness • Drowsiness • Dry mouth • Headache	• Lightheadedness • Liver toxicity (nefazodone) • Nervousness • Nausea	• Sustained erection or "priapism" (trazodone) • Vision problems • Weakness
Tricyclic antidepressants (TCAs)	• Amitriptyline (Elavil) • Amoxapine (Asendin) • Desipramine (Norpramin) • Doxepin (Sinequan) • Imipramine (Tofranil) • Nortriptyline (Pamelor) • Protriptyline (Vivactil) • Trimipramine (Surmontil)	• Abnormal heart rhythms • Bladder problems (urine retention) • Blurred vision • Confusion	• Constipation • Dry mouth • Fatigue, daytime drowsiness • Headache • Increased appetite, weight gain	• Insomnia • Low blood pressure • Muscle twitching • Sexual problems
Monoamine oxidase inhibitors (MAOIs)	• Isocarboxazid (Marplan) • Phenelzine (Nardil) • Selegiline (Emsam) • Tranylcypromine (Parnate)	• Drowsiness • Fast heartbeat • Headache • Insomnia	• Low or high blood pressure • Major interactions with certain foods and medications	• Nausea • Sexual problems

Selective serotonin reuptake inhibitors (SSRIs)

Selective serotonin reuptake inhibitors (SSRIs) are one of the newer antidepressant classes, and they are widely considered to be the first choice for patients who receive antidepressants. The first SSRI, fluoxetine (Prozac), appeared on the market in 1987. Since then, other drugs have joined Prozac, including citalopram (Celexa), sertraline (Zoloft), escitalopram (Lexapro) and paroxetine (Paxil). In January 2011, the FDA approved a new SSRI, vilazodone (Viibryd), which may have fewer sexual side effects than some of the other drugs in its class.

SSRIs block the return (reuptake) of serotonin to nerve cells, leaving higher levels of the neurotransmitter available to the brain. In addition to their antidepressant effects, SSRIs have other effects. In particular, they are very effective anti-anxiety medications that are now routinely used to treat anxiety conditions such as panic disorder and social anxiety disorder.

SSRIs can have side effects ranging from drowsiness to sexual problems. Women who are pregnant should use caution with any drug they take, including SSRIs. A trio of studies released in 2009 found that exposure to SSRIs and other antidepressants can have adverse effects on a baby's development. Babies who were exposed to antidepressants in the womb are more likely to have lower Apgar scores (a test used to assess the health of a newborn), slight delays in sitting and other developmental milestones, as well as one particular type of heart defect (although the overall risk of this defect is still low). But untreated depression during pregnancy and in the months after birth can also have negative effects on a baby's health. If you are depressed while pregnant, you should decide whether to use medications after carefully discussing the risks and benefits with a physician who is knowledgeable about the use of antidepressants during pregnancy.

SSRIs also can react with certain medications and supplements, including monoamine oxidase inhibitors (MAOIs) and St. John's wort. In addition, use SSRIs with caution if you are taking a blood thinner like warfarin (Coumadin) or medications that can increase the risk of stomach bleeding, such as high-dose nonsteroidal anti-inflammatory drugs (NSAIDS) like ibuprofen (Motrin) or aspirin or steroids such as prednisone.

Serotonin and norepinephrine reuptake inhibitors (SNRIs)

Serotonin and norepinephrine reuptake inhibitors (SNRIs) are another relatively new class of antidepressant, and they may be just as effective as the SSRIs. SNRIs work by altering levels of both serotonin and norepinephrine. Examples include duloxetine (Cymbalta), venlafaxine (Effexor) and desvenlafaxine (Pristiq). Some of the SNRIs are also approved for treatment of pain in such conditions as fibromyalgia. Therefore, particularly for individuals with both pain and depression, SNRIs may be prescribed as first-line antidepressants.

Norepinephrine-dopamine reuptake inhibitors (NDRIs)

Norepinephrine-dopamine reuptake inhibitors (NDRIs) increase the levels of both norepinephrine and dopamine in the brain. The only drug in this class is bupropion (Wellbutrin), but it is available in several different formulations, including a slow-release (Wellbutrin SR) and an extended-release (Wellbutrin XL) version, which only needs to be taken once a day. Although Wellbutrin is less likely to cause the sexual problems, weight gain and sedation of SSRIs and SNRIs, because it can slightly increase the risk for seizures, it is generally not recommended for people with seizure disorders or an increased risk for seizures (such as people with eating disorders or brain tumors).

Mirtazapine (Remeron)

Mirtazapine (Remeron) is an antidepressant that works by preventing neurotransmitters from binding with their nerve cell receptors. This effect increases the activity of norepinephrine and serotonin in the brain. Because mirtazapine tends to cause drowsiness and enhance appetite, it is sometimes considered an appealing option for depressed people who are struggling with insomnia or weight loss.

Reuptake inhibitors and receptor blockers

Reuptake inhibitors and receptor blockers work in two ways: they prevent the return of neurotransmitters to their receptors and they block nerve cell receptors. Two drugs in this class are FDA-approved to treat depression: trazodone (Desyrel) acts on serotonin and its receptors, and nefazodone (Serzone) blocks both serotonin and norepinephrine and their respective receptors. Like bupropion, trazodone and nefazodone are less likely to cause sexual dysfunction than the SSRIs or SNRIs. Like mirtazapine, they often help with insomnia. However, trazodone can cause an uncommon but well-documented side effect in men called priapism, or sustained erection, that requires immediate treatment if it lasts four or more hours. Nefazodone is rarely prescribed today because of its association with rare but serious liver problems.

Tricyclic antidepressants (TCAs)

Tricyclic antidepressants (TCAs) are among the oldest antidepressants. Drugs in this class include imipramine (Tofranil), nortriptyline (Pamelor), desipramine (Norpramin), amitriptyline (Elavil) and clomipramine (Anafranil). TCAs have been in use since the 1950s, but they're not the first choice for treating depression today because of their long list of side effects, which include weight gain, constipation, dry mouth, dizziness and heart conduction problems. TCAs also can worsen pre-existing conditions, such as narrow-angle glaucoma or an enlarged prostate. Recently, the company that makes one tricyclic antidepressant—desipramine—issued a warning for doctors to use extreme caution when prescribing the drug to patients with a family history of sudden death, abnormal heart rhythms or heart conduction disturbances. A large study in Scotland has also found that tricyclic antidepressants increase the risk of cardiovascular disease by 35 percent.

Because of tricyclic antidepressants' side effects, doctors usually don't turn to these drugs unless other medications have not been effective. But for some people who have not responded to newer antidepressants, these drugs can be lifesaving and they continue to be prescribed under special circumstances.

Monoamine oxidase inhibitors (MAOIs)

Monoamine oxidase inhibitors (MAOIs) work by preventing the enzyme monoamine oxidase from breaking down norepinephrine, serotonin and dopamine, leaving more of these neurotransmitters available in the brain. The MAOIs include tranylcypromine (Parnate), phenelzine (Nardil), isocarboxazid (Marplan) and selegiline (Emsam, which comes in a skin patch formulation). MAOIs are usually reserved for people who have not responded to other treatments because they can interact with certain aged and fermented foods, like aged cheeses, aged/smoked meats (including pepperoni), yeast extracts (such as Marmite) and certain alcoholic beverages such as ales and wine. Eating these foods while you're on an MAOI can lead to a sudden rise in blood pressure (hypertensive crisis), which requires emergency treatment.

A large number of medications can also cause life-threatening interactions with the MAOIs, including:

■ The painkiller meperidine (Demerol)

■ Virtually all of the other antidepressants

■ Other serotonin-acting medications, such as the migraine medications called "triptans"

If you have a mood disorder, anxiety or another condition in addition to your depression, your doctor may also prescribe one of the following medications:

■ Anti-anxiety medications—Also known as *anxiolytics*, anxiety-reducing drugs such as lorazepam (Ativan) or clonazepam (Klonopin) may be prescribed to treat anxiety, which often coexists with depression

■ Atypical antipsychotics—Aripiprazole (Abilify), quetiapine (Seroquel), or olanzapine (Zyprexa) may boost the effects of standard antidepressants in people with major depression and bipolar disorder

■ Mood stabilizers—Lithium and anticonvulsants such as valproic acid (Depakote), lamotrigine (Lamictal) and carbamazepine (Tegretol) are used to treat bipolar disorder

■ Adjunctive treatments—Other medications appear to help antidepressants work better in some people, but they still need more research. These medications include:

  • The anti-anxiety medication buspirone (Buspar)

  • A form of the thyroid hormone T3 (Cytomel)

  • Psychostimulants such as dextroamphetamine (Dexedrine), amphetamine salts (Adderall) or methylphenidate (Ritalin or Concerta)

  • Medications that stimulate dopamine receptors, such as pramipexole (Mirapex)

  • Medications used for narcolepsy, such as modafinil (Provigil)

  • Certain prescription forms of the B vitamin folate, which are available as L-methylfolate (Deplin) or folinic acid (Leucovorin)

Your doctor will choose a medication based on your symptoms, how well you can tolerate the drug's reported side effects, and its cost (taking into account what your insurance company will or will not cover).

Unfortunately, the first medication you take may not whisk away your depression. Only about one-third of people with depression improve completely with the first medication they take. For others, it takes some thoughtful trial and error. Your doctor will adjust the dosage or change the medication over a six- to 12-week period until you find the drug and dose that work best for you. In some cases, two or more drugs may be necessary to give you the best possible relief.

New depression treatment guidelines from the American Psychiatric Association recommend that doctors use maintenance drug therapy to prevent depression from returning. This is especially important for people whose depression tends to recur, and particularly for those who have had three or more episodes of depression or chronic illness.

In a few cases, medication may not be the best option. If you have mild, short-term depression, research finds that the benefits of antidepressants are limited. Only patients who scored 25 or higher on the Hamilton Rating Scale for Depression (which indicates severe depression) benefitted more from taking an antidepressant medication than from a placebo (sugar pill). The study questions whether people with mild or moderate depression might be better off starting with other treatments, such as psychotherapy. However, for people with mild depression who had severe depression in the past, or for those whose depression has been going on for many months or years, medications remain an important option.

Remember that any of the drugs used to treat depression can have side effects. Your doctor should go over all of the potential side effects with you when the drug is prescribed and should document any side effects you do experience in your medical record. Side effects often go unreported because many patients neglect to tell their doctors about the symptoms they are experiencing. In fact, researchers have found that patients may experience up to 20 times more side effects than their psychiatrists recorded. It is very important that you share information about side effects because your doctor may need to lower the dosage or switch you to a new medication. And remember that stopping antidepressants on your own is never a good idea; discontinuation of medications not only leaves your depression untreated it may trigger its own side effects such as nausea, headaches, muscle aches and more intense depression. Children may also be treated with antidepressants, but doctors need to be cautious when prescribing medication to their younger patients. Concerns over the use of antidepressants in children and adolescents arose after a study suggested that antidepressants cause or worsen suicidal thoughts in this age group. Although the risk was still relatively small (4 percent in the antidepressant group, compared with 2 percent in children taking a sugar pill), in October 2004 the U.S.

Food and Drug Administration began requiring manufacturers to label all antidepressants with a strong "black box" warning about the risk of suicidal thoughts and behaviors in children. A study in the April 2012 issue of the journal *Pediatrics* found that all antidepressants cause a similar suicide risk in children. The authors say doctors should be very careful about monitoring their young patients who take these medications.

That doesn't mean parents shouldn't consider antidepressants for their children, only that the risks of these drugs need to be weighed very carefully against the benefits. Currently, Prozac is the only antidepressant approved for use in children ages 8 and older. The SSRI Lexapro is FDA-approved for the treatment of depression in adolescents. Other antidepressants, including Zoloft, Luvox and Anafranil are used off-label in children, even though they have not specifically been approved for that age group. The FDA recommends that children with major depression not be treated with Paxil.

Psychotherapy

Another important component of treatment for depression is to talk out the issues that may be causing or worsening your symptoms with a trained professional. It might sound simple, but talking can lift a lot of the emotional weight that you feel. And talk therapy doesn't simply mean "venting." Talk therapy (called psychotherapy or just "therapy") will help you identify the problems that are causing your depression so that you can begin to work through those problems. Increasingly, talk therapy also involves learning specific coping skills and problem-solving strategies.

Individual, Family and Group Counseling

Therapy for depression is individualized. While one person might benefit from one-on-one time with his or her therapist, another might feel more comfortable discussing issues in a supportive group setting. These individual preferences are why counseling comes in several different forms.

■ Individual therapy: You meet alone with a therapist.

■ Group therapy: You meet with several other patients. Sometimes the group will focus on a particular issue, such as domestic abuse, substance abuse or bereavement. A therapist will facilitate the group, introducing topics for discussion and directing the meetings. The benefit of having other people at your therapy session is that it gives you the opportunity to learn from people who have gone through the same issues. Being with a group of people in a similar situation also can make you feel like you're not alone. The downside is that you will have to be willing to share very personal thoughts and experiences in a group setting.

■ Couples and family therapy: Your spouse, parents and/or children will accompany you to the session. During meetings with the therapist, you will work together to improve communication and resolve any relationship issues you are experiencing.

Cognitive Behavioral Therapy (CBT)

Imagine this scenario: You're on your way to a cocktail party and you get stuck in traffic. Immediately you think, "I'm going to be late, and the host is going to be furious with me." That thought is followed by, "I'm late for everything. I'm such a failure." When you arrive at the party a few minutes late and see that the other guests are already deep in conversation, you think, "They're all ignoring me. They must hate me." After all of those negative thoughts, how much do you think you're going to enjoy the party?

People with depression are often plagued by these kinds of negative thoughts. The idea behind cognitive behavioral therapy (CBT) is that your thoughts can have a big impact on your mood. This treatment aims to identify and then change your negative perceptions to give you a more positive outlook.

CBT starts with identifying the negative thoughts you have about yourself ("I'm a failure"), your environment ("Everyone hates me") and your future ("I have nothing to look forward to"). Working closely with your therapist, you start to understand how certain negative beliefs have no basis in reality. Then, you reframe those false beliefs and replace them with more positive ones. CBT is typically meant to be a fairly short-term treatment, lasting a few weeks or months.

Studies have shown that CBT is very effective for depression—as effective as antidepressant medications in many cases. Some research indicates that combining CBT with medication makes treatment even more effective, particularly for people with major depression. It may also help prevent depression that has been treated from returning.

Usually CBT is done one-on-one in an office with a therapist, but new technologies can make CBT available from your own living room using a telephone or computer. Read the section on accessing care on page 65 to learn more.

An intriguing new form of psychotherapy, which uses many of the principles of CBT is known as concreteness training (Box 5-2).

Interpersonal Therapy (IPT)

Relationships can play a very important part in triggering depression. When your marriage is on the rocks or you're struggling with the stress of an abusive family member or boss, it's hard to keep a positive mood.

Interpersonal therapy focuses on identifying the relationship issues that are driving your depression symptoms, particularly unresolved grief, relationship conflicts, transitions to a new role (such as from wife to wife and mother) and difficulty with interpersonal relationships. Then it helps you improve your communication and conflict resolution skills so that you are better equipped to handle issues that arise with your friends and family members.

As with CBT, interpersonal therapy is used over the short-term. You will typically have 12 to 16 treatment sessions, which focus on first identifying problems and then teaching you how to resolve them. Interpersonal therapy works well for people with mild-to-moderate depression, and it may be used together with antidepressants.

Psychodynamic Therapy

Psychodynamic therapy is often a longer-term approach to treating depression. This treatment seeks to identify the roots of your depression by focusing on the behaviors and relationships that are making you unhappy and then developing new insights about how they affect you. You may go back as far as your childhood, recalling events that you might have consciously forgotten but which are unconsciously driving your dark mood. For example, it might be that your mother was particularly critical of you as a child, and now you have turned that critical eye on yourself. By using techniques such as self-reflection and self-examination, your therapist can bring the painful memories and feelings that are haunting you to light and then try to work through them so you can learn how to live a healthier, happier life.

An analysis of several studies published by the American Psychological Association found psychodynamic therapy to be effective for treating depression as well as anxiety and other co-existing conditions. What's more, the benefits of psychodynamic therapy continue even after treatment has ended.

Because psychodynamic therapy tends to be more open-ended and longer-term than CBT or IPT, it may not be as efficient for treating depression in some people. However, shorter-term and more focused versions of psychodynamic therapy are being developed that may work better in these patients.

Dialectical Behavior Therapy (DBT)

Dialectical Behavior Therapy (DBT) is similar to CBT and IPT, and it is practiced in both individual and group settings. DBT was primarily developed for people who struggle with a particularly severe form of personality disorder called borderline personality disorder, which includes profound feelings of emptiness, unstable interpersonal relationships, self-destructive behaviors and suicidal tendencies. DBT emphasizes acceptance and change, which was influenced by psychological research and practice as well as by Buddhism. In recent years, DBT has been used with some success to treat people who do not necessarily have borderline personality disorder but who are dealing with chronic unhappiness and thoughts of suicide.

Brain Stimulation Therapies

No one is exactly sure why, but it appears that stimulating the brain, certain parts of the brain or specific major nerves can sometimes produce relief from depression, even when other therapies fail. Different brain stimulation therapies vary with respect to the area being stimulated, the source of the stimulation and the invasiveness of the procedure, but in all cases the goal is to get brain cells firing.

Electroconvulsive Therapy

The thought of getting an electric shock to the brain might sound pretty extreme. Thanks to movie depictions such as Jack Nicholson's harrowing ordeal in the film *One Flew Over the Cuckoo's Nest*, many people picture patients getting strapped to a table and writhing in agony as shocks course through their bodies.

In reality, electroconvulsive therapy (ECT) is a safe and highly effective medical therapy used to treat severe depression that has not responded well enough to medication and psychotherapy. There is a lot of evidence to show that ECT is an effective treatment for people who don't respond to many different types of antidepressants. Sometimes

ECT is used before medications or psychotherapy in people with severe and life-threatening symptoms that require a more fast-acting treatment.

ECT does use an electrical shock to trigger seizures in the brain, but the current is well-controlled and delivered while the patient is under anesthesia, making it painless. It's designed to cause the brain to release the neurotransmitters that improve mood.

If your doctor decides that you're a good candidate for ECT, you will have the treatment done at a hospital, either as an outpatient or with an overnight stay. ECT is given up to three or four times a week, for about eight to 12 sessions overall. Usually both an anesthesiologist and a psychiatrist who are trained in ECT will supervise your treatment.

Before the treatment, you will receive an anesthetic through a vein (IV). You'll also receive a muscle relaxant so that your body remains calm during the procedure. Once you are asleep, electrodes will be placed on your head and a small amount of electrical current will be delivered to your brain. That shock will cause you to have a controlled seizure that will last from 20 seconds to one minute. After you wake up, you'll have some time to recover and then you can go home.

Some people experience side effects from the anesthesia or from the ECT itself, such as confusion, short-term memory loss, nausea or headache. Blood pressure and heart rhythm sometimes can be affected.

Studies find that ECT is highly effective, and it starts to work quickly—within days or weeks. About 80 percent of patients who have the treatment report that their depression is either gone or significantly reduced. Most patients who respond to ECT receive a follow-up antidepressant to prevent relapse of depression. Some people who do not respond well to medications benefit from ongoing "maintenance" ECT, usually about one or two sessions per month, to stave off depression.

Vagus Nerve Stimulation

In vagus nerve stimulation (VNS), a pacemaker-like device called a pulse generator (which is about the size of a silver dollar) is implanted in the chest by a surgeon (usually a neurosurgeon or thoracic surgeon). The pulse generator sends signals to the vagus nerve in the neck for about 30 seconds once every five minutes. These signals are thought to improve mood, although doctors still don't know exactly how the technique works to improve symptoms of depression.

Although VNS has been FDA-approved since the late 1990s for treating epilepsy, and more recently it has been FDA-approved for treatment-resistant depression, its use for depression is still somewhat controversial. Evidence is mixed as to whether it really works. Because implanting the pulse generator requires surgery, risks can include infection, bleeding, pain, hoarseness, cough and damage to the vagus nerve. Even after VNS, many patients need to continue depression treatments such as medication and therapy.

Deep Brain Stimulation

A similar technique, called deep brain stimulation (DBS), also involves implanting a device in the chest. This time, however, the device is connected by wires to electrodes implanted deep in the brain in order to send electrical signals directly there. These signals stimulate areas in the brain that affect mood and depression. As with VNS, risks of DBS include bleeding and infection at the site of the incision. Implanting the electrodes in the brain can also trigger bleeding in the brain or even a stroke. Recent research has demonstrated the benefits of DBS for treatment-resistant depression as well as depression associated with bipolar disorder (Box 5-3).

Transcranial Magnetic Stimulation

Another new brain stimulation technique, called transcranial magnetic stimulation (TMS), has generated a lot of interest in the medical community because it involves no surgery and few risks, and there is mounting evidence of its effectiveness. This noninvasive therapy, which received FDA approval in 2008, uses an electromagnetic coil to send pulses to a part of the brain that helps regulate mood. Unlike more invasive brain stimulation techniques, TMS can be delivered right in a doctor's office with specialized equipment. Studies are demonstrating that TMS can benefit many people with major depression (Box 5-4).

TMS has its downsides, though. Currently, many insurance companies do not cover the costs of TMS, which are prohibitive for many patients. The currently approved technology for TMS may not be as effective as ECT, which is why ECT remains the treatment of choice for severe depression that has not responded to medication and psychotherapy.

Transcranial Direct Current Stimulation

An even newer brain stimulation technique is called transcranial direct current stimulation (tDCS). Also noninvasive, this technique involves using electrodes placed on the scalp to run a weak electrical current into the front portion of the brain (Box 5-5).

Trigeminal Nerve Stimulation

Another new electrical stimulation therapy, also requiring further study, and also showing promise for treating depression is called trigeminal nerve stimulation (TNS). This therapy was originally designed for patients with treatment-resistant epilepsy. TNS uses a stimulator about the size of a large cell phone, which is connected by wires to electrodes attached to the forehead. The electrodes send an electrical current to the trigeminal nerve in the face.

Stimulating this nerve sends signals deep into the brain in a noninvasive way, researchers say. A study reported that 80 percent of patients achieved remission with TNS, and the TNS technique didn't have any side effects. These results are still preliminary, however. Much more work is needed before TNS can be used in patients with depression.

New Treatments for Depression

Researchers are constantly working to fine-tune and add to the currently available therapies for depression. Here are a few of the exciting new developments you might expect to see in the near future:

Agomelatine (Valdoxan)

Clinical trials are under way in the United States to study an antidepressant that was first developed in Europe. Valdoxan works on two types of receptors: a type of serotonin receptor called 5HT2C as well as a receptor for the natural sleep-regulating hormone, melatonin (Box 5-6).

Triple reuptake inhibitors

Researchers are working on a number of antidepressants that block the reuptake of three neurotransmitters: serotonin, norepinephrine and dopamine. They hope that by making more of all three of these chemicals available to the brain, triple reuptake inhibitors will have a more significant impact on depression than the antidepressants that are currently available (which generally work on only one or two neurotransmitters).

Glutamate blocking antidepressants

Glutamate is a neurotransmitter that is produced by neurons and other brain cells called glia. Even though it is a naturally occurring neurotransmitter, glutamate can have toxic effects on brain cells when it is produced in larger-than-normal amounts.

There are a variety of receptors for glutamate, and a number of medications block these receptors. These include the anesthetic ketamine and the medication riluzole used to treat ALS (amyotrophic lateral sclerosis, also called Lou Gehrig's disease). In recent years, research has suggested that these medications may also be useful in the treatment of depression. A number of clinical trials are looking at whether medications that act on the glutamate system may represent a brand new class of antidepressant medications.

Stress hormone blocking agents

Certain hormones released during the "fight or flight" stress response (such as cortisol) may have a role in depression, particularly in forms of depression that develop from chronic stress. Medications such as mifepristone (Mifeprex), which block cortisol production, are currently being investigated for the treatment of depression. Drugs such as these may someday help relieve depression symptoms or reduce the risk of developing depression following stressful life events.

Brain-derived neurotrophic factor

It is now believed that many antidepressants boost the levels or activity of chemicals in the brain that promote nerve health and growth, such as brain-derived neurotrophic factor (BDNF). Some researchers believe that antidepressants may reduce the risk of brain atrophy (shrinkage) in patients with chronic depression because they can promote BDNF. Although BDNF cannot be given as pills, the observation that antidepressants may have an effect on BDNF has opened new avenues for treatments that replicate this action on the brain.

Fast-acting ketamine

A new, fast-acting form of an antidepressant that has already been shown to be effective for treating severely depressed patients is under development. Ketamine has been used as a general anesthetic for children, but a few years ago doctors found that the drug, when administered in lower doses, also benefits patients with depression. In initial clinical studies, 70 percent of patients who were resistant to other antidepressants showed improvements—not in weeks or months like with other antidepressants—but within hours of being given the drug.

Yale University scientists think they've discovered the reason why the drug works so quickly. In rats, ketamine doesn't just improve depression symptoms, it actually restores connections between neurons that have been damaged by long-term stress. New research also highlights the benefits of fast-acting ketamine for depression associated with bipolar disorder (Box 5-7).

Despite its apparent benefits, fast-acting ketamine isn't going to be available to consumers just yet. It is challenging to administer because it has to be delivered intravenously, and in some cases it can cause psychotic side effects. In addition, most people who respond to ketamine do not sustain the response and still need to be treated with other modalities including standard antidepressants and psychotherapy to maintain remission.

NSI-189

An investigational drug that is so new it doesn't even have a proper name is currently known as NSI-189. This drug works like no other. It actually stimulates the growth of new neurons within the brain, particularly within the hippocampus, an area that has been implicated in depression.

While not yet available to the public, NSI-189 has been approved by the FDA for testing in patients with depression.

Natural and Alternative Therapies

Some people prefer to try alternative therapies for depression. Although some of these treatments have shown effectiveness against depression symptoms, they may not be enough to treat the condition, particularly if you have more severe depression. It's important to check with your doctor before taking any therapy—even a natural remedy—to make sure you are receiving the best and safest treatment possible.

A number of herbal (plant-based) and non-herbal supplements have been suggested for treating depression. Although the labels of these supplements may boast that they are "natural," use caution. The FDA does not regulate supplements as it does medications, so it's hard to know exactly what you're getting when you buy a bottle, or whether the supplement will actually work. Any supplement has the potential to cause side effects, and it may interact with other medications you are taking. Check with your doctor before trying any of the following alternative depression remedies:

Omega-3 fatty acid supplements

The essential polyunsaturated fatty acids found in fish like salmon, tuna and halibut, as well as in flaxseed and other plants are crucial to healthy brain function. A number of studies have found that people with diets that are high in fish are less likely to be depressed. Results of studies on the effectiveness of omega-3 fatty acid supplements for treating depression have been mixed (Box 5-8), but because of the overall health benefits, experts say it makes sense to add foods that are rich in omega-3 fatty acids to your diet. For people who do not eat fish, some studies suggest that low doses (about 1 mg/day) of omega-3 fatty acid supplements may have an antidepressant benefit, particularly when added to standard antidepressant treatment regimens.

S-adenosylmethionine (SAMe)

S-adenosylmethionine or SAMe (pronounced "Sammy") is a natural substance found in all of the body's cells. It helps produce serotonin and dopamine, and it participates in myriad other natural physiological reactions in the body. Taking SAMe in supplement form is thought to increase the levels of certain brain chemicals and improve mood.

Studies that were conducted in Europe with an injected form of SAMe showed that the supplement was similar in effectiveness to low doses of tricyclic antidepressants. A study showed that high doses of oral SAMe along with usual antidepressants benefitted depressed adults who had failed to respond to standard treatment. More research is needed to determine the safety and effectiveness of SAMe. A concern with the product is that SAMe appears to worsen or even bring out mania in depressed people who have bipolar disorder.

St. John's Wort

This flower extract is one of the most popular, and best studied, alternative remedies for depression. Although a large review of studies conducted by the National Center for Complementary and Alternative Medicine (NCCAM) showed that the herb wasn't any better for treating major depression than a placebo, it may be more effective for mild-to-moderate depression. St. John's wort can cause side effects, including fatigue, increased blood pressure, sensitivity to sunlight and stomach upset. It also can interact with certain medications, including immune suppressing drugs such as cyclosporine, HIV medications, asthma medications, digoxin, oral contraceptives and blood thinners. If you are considering using St. John's wort, weigh the risks carefully with your doctor.

B Vitamins

There is some evidence linking low levels of certain B vitamins, such as vitamin B12 and folate, with depression. These vitamins are important for the production of brain chemicals that help regulate mood. At least in older people, researchers have found that higher intake of some B vitamins may help prevent depression. Seniors are prone to vitamin B deficiency because they are more likely to have medical conditions that interfere with the proper absorption of these nutrients. A study found that, for each additional 10 mg of vitamin B6, and 10 micrograms of vitamin B12 that seniors consumed from both food and supplements, the odds of having depression symptoms dropped by 2 percent. Several studies have shown that adding folate in different forms including folic acid, L-methylfolate and folinic acid may boost the effectiveness of standard antidepressants.

You can ask your doctor for a blood test that will determine whether your B vitamin levels are low. If they are, that increases the likelihood that supplementing with B vitamins will help your depression.

Therapies

In addition to herbal and non-herbal natural remedies, several complementary and integrative therapies can be used with traditional depression treatments. Depending on the severity of your depression and its symptoms, you may wish to discuss these treatments with your doctor. Whenever a treatment is used for depression that has not yet been well established, it is particularly important to monitor its effectiveness. If the remedy does not work quickly enough, your doctor can prescribe a treatment that is known to be effective.

Here is the evidence on a few popular alternative therapies for depression:

Massage

If you have ever had a massage, you know how relaxed the therapy can make you feel. A review of studies found that massage might actually help relieve the symptoms of depression. The studies included in the review found that massage therapy had "potentially significant effects" on the symptoms of depression, possibly through its ability to reduce stress and induce a state of relaxation.

Acupuncture

This traditional Chinese medicine practice of stimulating various pressure points throughout the body with very fine needles has been used to treat conditions ranging from osteoarthritis to low back pain. Although one review of studies did not find enough evidence to recommend the use of acupuncture for depression, a study found that acupuncture significantly improved depression in pregnant women. Acupuncture is generally very safe. If any side effects occur, they are usually very mild. Infection can be spread with acupuncture if needles are not properly sterilized, however. So, if you decide to try this therapy, make sure your practitioner uses disposable needles or properly sterilizes reusable needles.

Relaxation Techniques

Guided imagery, in which you use tapes or the help of an instructor to focus on a particular image (such as a lemon) in great detail, can be a good way to teach your body how to relax. Meditation, in which you sit quietly for 10 to 15 minutes and repeat a word or "mantra", is another effective relaxation technique. Yoga can also help relax the body and mind. A number of formal talk therapies (psychotherapies) such as cognitive behavioral therapy, dialectical behavior therapy and mindfulness-based cognitive therapy have adapted elements of these methods into their treatments.

Light therapy

Anyone who has been outside on a sunny day knows that sunlight can really boost mood, and research is confirming this effect. In people with seasonal affective disorder (SAD), long, dark winter days trigger depression. These symptoms are thought to be caused by alterations in the body's circadian rhythm and production of melatonin (a hormone that regulates sleep and mood). Light therapy can help regulate circadian rhythms and melatonin production to boost mood not only in people with SAD but also in those with depression who want to try an alternative to medication and therapy.

During light therapy, you sit in front of a special light box (don't try this with any old table lamp—it won't work). At a dose of 10,000 lux (a measure of brightness), the light is brighter than typical indoor lighting but not quite as bright as sunlight. Starting with 15-minute sessions, you gradually increase the time to anywhere from 30 minutes to two hours. Light therapy is usually most effective when done first thing in the morning. If you do it at night, the therapy might interfere with your sleep. Other side effects may include headache, eye strain and mild irritability.

Staying Healthy

Depression can sap your will to take care of yourself, but more and more research is showing that poor diet and lack of physical activity can lead to or worsen depression while getting moving and eating healthy can be an important, even crucial, component of getting better.

Exercise

Just about everyone knows that exercise is good for your body. Getting in a good daily workout not only helps control your weight, but it can also prevent conditions like diabetes, high blood pressure and heart disease. Research is revealing that what's good for the body is also good for the mind. When you go for a run or a swim, your brain releases brain chemicals such as norepinephrine and endorphins—both of which can boost mood (if you've ever heard the expression, "runner's high," it refers to the feeling runners get from these chemicals).

Working out regularly will also help you look your best, which can have a big impact on your self-esteem, and it can keep your mind off of what's troubling you. In fact, preliminary research finds that exercise might be as effective for relieving depression as antidepressants, and its benefits may last over the long-term.

Any exercise can work, so pick something you enjoy, whether it's step aerobics or dancing. For seniors, tai chi appears to be an effective way to battle the blues. If you're too busy to spend an hour at the gym each day, sneak 10- to 15-minute bursts of exercise into your day. Even housework and gardening count as exercise. Just be sure to get in a total of 30 to 60 minutes of physical activity on most, if not all days of the week.

If you are using exercise to treat depression, work closely with your primary care doctor or a mental health professional to design an exercise regimen that is achievable for you. If brushing your teeth in the morning or getting dressed already feels like too much of an effort, even minimal exercise is going to be too much for you until you can get your depression under control with other treatments. As you begin to feel better, you can gradually incorporate exercise into your treatment plan. It may even help your medications or psychotherapy work better.

Diet

What you eat can have a big impact on your mood. Foods like fish, nuts and seeds, which are high in omega-3 fatty acids, may help ward off depression. That might be why people who eat a Mediterranean diet (in which olive oil, nuts and fish are staples) are less likely to develop depression than people who eat other kinds of diets. Processed and sugary foods are high in simple carbs and trans fats, which may boost energy transiently, but ultimately can drain your energy and make you feel even more down in the dumps. Yet often these are the very foods people crave when they are depressed. If you've ever grabbed a chocolate bar when you were feeling down, you're not alone. Research finds that both women and men tend to eat more chocolate when they're depressed.

Accessing Care

As mentioned previously, about half of depressed people do not receive the care they need. There are several barriers to receiving care, including the inability to physically get to the places where care is available, cost issues and the stigma or discomfort associated with entering therapy.

Fortunately, some pretty innovative yet simple technological tools are helping to surmount some of these barriers. For instance, researchers out of the University of Aukland in New Zealand have developed an interactive 3D fantasy game designed to help adolescents work through their symptoms of depression (Box 5-9). Hopefully with time, inexpensive and widely available technologies like cell phones and the Internet will provide more widespread, affordable access to care for depression and also help lift some of the psychological barriers to accepting help.

When Depression Treatments Don't Work

Your doctor will work closely with you to find the best treatment, whether that is medication, psychotherapy or a combination of therapies. But depression can be a tough target to nail. You might have to experiment with several different treatments before you find the one that works best for you. Your doctor may need to adjust your antidepressant dose, switch you to a new medication, combine medications or psychotherapies or add a technique like brain stimulation if medication and therapy aren't enough. You can also discuss alternative and integrative therapies for depression, such as exercise or acupuncture.

If it seems as though you've tried every medicine and therapy and your depression still refuses to go away, you might have treatment-resistant depression, which is the term for depression that hasn't responded to several different antidepressants or psychotherapy. This doesn't mean that you'll never find a treatment that works, or that you'll be forced to endure depression for the rest of your life. It just means that you and your doctor will have to try a few different approaches to relieve your depression.

Know that there will be a therapy out there that will eventually work for you. Don't give up. Recent research has shown that most people who are depressed need to try several therapies—or combinations of therapies—before they find the regimen that works for them. In other words, it's quite normal not to feel better right away, but most people who persevere eventually find a treatment that works. Moreover, people who do find the treatment that works well for them are less likely to have a relapse of their depression in the future. While you are working with your doctor to find the right treatment, use the next chapter to make sure that you have the support you need from friends, family members and professionals. ■

6 LIVING WITH DEPRESSION

When you have depression, it's almost impossible to see the light at the end of the tunnel. Without hope and a belief that your sadness will ultimately lift, it's tempting to curl up under your covers and hide from the world or even begin to contemplate suicide as the only way out.

Don't give up. There is an end to your depression. Whether it comes in the form of medication, therapy, alternative treatments or a combination of all three, recovery is possible. You can beat your depression. So many others in your situation already have.

Know that you don't have to and in fact should not even try to do this alone. Too much solitude has been linked with depression risk (Box 6-1). There are many people out there who can help you: Family members and friends who love you, trained professionals who know how to get you the treatment you need and millions of other people who have been in the exact same situation you're experiencing now. In this chapter, you'll learn how to find the support you need. You'll also learn how to offer your support if it is not you but a friend or loved one who is dealing with depression.

Finding Support

Getting help for your depression starts with a visit to your doctor or a mental health professional for diagnosis and treatment. Once treatment is under way, seek out the type of support that works for you, whether it is:

■ Talking to a friend or family member

■ Meeting with a therapist or counselor for personal, marriage, family or group therapy

■ Joining a support group of people with depression

■ Visiting an online support group

■ Talking to a trusted member of your church, synagogue, mosque or other religious organization

The organizations listed in Appendix II are wonderful resources. They can provide you with background information about depression and the latest treatments for it. Many can also point you to doctors and support groups in your area. Most people begin to get relief simply by

> *A human being can survive almost anything, as long as she sees the end in sight. But depression is so insidious, and it compounds daily, that it's impossible to ever see the end. The fog is like a cage without a key.*
>
> —Elizabeth Wurtzel, author of *Prozac Nation*

NEW FINDING

Box 6-1: Living alone can give you the blues

Human beings are social animals, so it may come as no surprise that living alone has been identified as a risk factor for depression. For research published in the March 2012 issue of *BMC Public Health*, investigators looked at data collected on more than 3,500 men and women who provided information about their lifestyle and health-related habits. The investigators found that those who live alone are 80 percent more likely to purchase antidepressants than those living with others. The researchers also noted that since the most isolated people are the least likely to participate in such a study, these results may actually underestimate the impact of living alone and/or social isolation on depression risk.

sharing their burden with people who care about them, who have special expertise in evaluating and treating depression, or who know from their own personal experience about living with depression. Because it can take weeks or even months to recover from depression, it is well worth taking the time to find the support you need to get you safely through this challenging period in your life.

Helping a Friend or Loved One With Depression

You might have picked up this report not for yourself but for a friend or family member who you suspect has depression. Read through the symptoms in Chapter 4 and see if they match with what your loved one is experiencing. If the symptoms do seem similar, it's time to step in and offer your help.

Despite your best intentions, helping someone with depression isn't always easy. Your friend might not realize he or she is depressed or may not be willing to accept your help. Realize that you cannot "cure" that person, no matter how hard you try. All you can do is help someone recognize that there is a problem, let him or her know you care, and suggest professional help.

When you first approach your friend or loved one about depression, bring with you a few recommendations for available local services, such as the names and phone numbers of therapists or support groups. Gently keep track of whether your loved one seeks treatment and takes medication as prescribed. Offer your encouragement along the way. Be on the lookout for the signs of suicidal tendencies listed at the end of this chapter. If you see any of these warning signs, call a mental health professional or 911 right away.

Don't shy away from asking someone directly about depression. Even trained professionals sometimes don't recognize the signs and symptoms in themselves. Feedback from a concerned friend or family member is often a helpful "wake-up call," whether or not that friend or family member decides to act on it right away. Similarly, don't hesitate to ask whether a close friend or family member has had any thoughts of self-harm or not wanting to live. Asking about suicide does not make it more likely. On the contrary, it allows a loved one to share the burden and get the help he or she needs. Suicidal thoughts are often part of being depressed. They do not necessarily require hospitalization, but they do need to be taken seriously, and they always require urgent evaluation.

Preventing Episodes of Depression

Depression is not like chickenpox or polio. You can't take a vaccine to ward off the blues. Sometimes depression can't be prevented. But you can lessen the blow of depression by recognizing when you have symptoms and getting professional help. Here are a few other tips to help relieve the depression you are feeling and possibly prevent future episodes.

Follow the treatment plan your doctor prescribed. Contact your doctor right away if you are having bothersome or worrisome side effects from your medication. Keep in mind that some side effects get better on their own within the first few days of starting a medication, while others require a change in dose or medication. Don't change any part of your treatment without first talking to your doctor.

Keep your long-term goals in mind. It usually takes two to three weeks before you begin to feel better, and it can take as long as six to 12 weeks to know whether a medication will be fully effective for you. Stopping and starting medications prematurely will not give your body enough time to respond to the recommended treatment, and it won't allow your doctor to determine whether the medication is right for you.

Take it easy on yourself, but avoid too much undeserved self-praise (Box 6-2). It's easy to blame yourself for the way you feel, or to think that you deserve to feel the way that you do. Even if you have made some bad choices in life, remember that virtually everyone has made bad choices at times and yet not everyone experiences depression. The worst time to evaluate your decisions or actions is while you are in the midst of depression, when you are more likely than ever to be your harshest critic. What you're experiencing is a medical condition that needs to be treated. Excessive feelings of guilt or self-blame are symptoms of your disease, not evidence of your poor character. It is best to wait until after your depression is treated and your thinking is clearer to reassess your life and the choices you've made.

Take care of yourself

Incorporate the following healthy lifestyle choices, many of which have been shown to have a big impact on depression:

Box 6-2: Too much self-praise may actually contribute to depression

We live in a culture where self-congratulatory behavior is encouraged. Managed to graduate from preschool? Let's throw a party! Cut down your coffee consumption from eight down to just seven cups a day? You're a model of self-restraint! But new research suggests that congratulating ourselves without just cause may actually backfire and leave us feeling dejected.

For research published in the October 2011 issue of *Emotion*, investigators out of the University of Pennsylvania conducted two different experiments with thousands of high school and college students in the U.S. and Hong Kong. In the first experiment, the students completed an academic exam and were asked to rate their performance compared with other students at their schools. Subsequently, the students completed questionnaires about feelings of depression. In the second experiment, the researchers gave feedback to undergraduates about exercises they completed that made high performers believe they had performed poorly and low performers believe they had performed well.

Results of both experiments revealed that those who rated their performance as significantly greater than it actually was were more likely to feel dejected. Those who performed just as poorly but who had also correctly rated their performance as poor had no such negative reaction. The experts speculate that unjustified self-praise can backfire when one's true talents (or lack thereof) are revealed or because it acts as a barrier to self-improvement. Interestingly, the researchers also found that the Asian students, by and large, were more humble than their American counterparts. That is, they were less likely to overrate their performance and therefore less likely to feel dejected.

NEW FINDING

Box 6-3: Relieving depression may be a walk in the park

The benefits of staying active as a means of warding off or relieving depression have been demonstrated in several studies. But new research suggests that choosing a pleasant, natural environment for your exercise may provide additional benefits. In research published online in May 2012 ahead of print in the *Journal of Affective Disorders*, 20 adults with clinical depression walked for an hour in a woodland park or in a traffic-heavy downtown region. All participants were asked to think about a personal experience that was painful and unresolved. After their walk, the participants completed a series of mental tests designed to assess their attention, memory and mood. A week later, the participants repeated the exercise, except this time those who walked in the city switched to the wooded area and those who walked in the wooded area switched to the city. Both walks helped lift the participants' moods. But walking in the wooded area was also associated with a 16 percent increase in attention and working memory, both of which are frequently adversely affected by depression. No such effect was seen when the participants walked in the city

NEW FINDING

Box 6-4: Poor diet could give you the blues

Typical advice for depressed individuals is to maintain a healthy lifestyle, and eating right is an important component of that. Now research is providing concrete evidence about why avoiding junk food is particularly important for those who are depressed.

A study published online in the January 2011 issue of *PLoS One* finds that a diet high in trans fats, an unhealthy type of fat found in many packaged and processed foods, could increase the risk of depression by nearly 50 percent. The study included more than 12,000 people who agreed to have their diet, lifestyle and health analyzed. People who ate a lot of fast food and other trans fat-laden foods were up to 48 percent more likely to be depressed compared to participants who didn't eat trans fats. The more trans fats people ate, the greater their risk for depression became. People who ate healthy polyunsaturated fats (found in fish and vegetable oils), on the other hand, had a lower risk for depression.

More recently, Spanish researchers published a study in the April 2012 issue of the journal *Public Health Nutrition* revealing that eaters of fast food, such as pizza, hamburgers and hot dogs, were 51 percent more likely to develop depression than those who rarely or never indulged in these foods. A similar link was found among eaters of commercially baked goods, such as cakes, croissants and doughnuts

Exercise for 30 to 60 minutes a day

When you work out, your body releases endorphins—chemicals that make you feel better. Research has found that exercising for 30 minutes a day can be just as effective at relieving the symptoms of major depression as drug therapy. Exercising will also keep your body in shape, boosting your self-esteem. Even something as simple as a walk in the park can help boost your mood (Box 6-3).

Maintain a healthy diet

Research shows that a healthy diet can help ward off depression and vice versa (Box 6-4). Limit unhealthy fats and sugars and instead eat plenty of fruits, vegetables, fish and whole grains. Avoid alcohol and drugs. Depression treatments don't work as well with even moderate use of alcohol or recreational drugs such as marijuana or cocaine. Abstinence is best when you are embarking on a course of antidepressant treatment. If you cannot simply taper off alcohol and drug use, get treated for alcohol/drug problems while you are being evaluated and treated for depression. When depression coincides with alcohol and other drug problems, mental health and addiction professionals can work collaboratively to treat both issues.

Sleep well

Depression and poor sleep are closely linked. Understandably, people who are depressed can have trouble getting to sleep or staying asleep because of the persistent worries that plague them. When you don't sleep well, you feel worse during the day. You have less energy to go out with friends or exercise. A lack of sleep exacerbates the depression you're already experiencing. A study in published in the journal *Sleep* linked poor sleep with depression and suicidal thoughts in adolescents. Adolescents in the study who went to bed at midnight or later had an increased risk for depression and suicidal thoughts compared to those who maintained a bedtime of 10 p.m. or earlier. The authors say a lack of sleep could contribute to depression in part by making it difficult for kids to deal with daily life stresses.

To make sure you're getting enough sleep, practice good "sleep hygiene" (Box 6-5). Some people have sleep disorders such as obstructive sleep apnea or restless legs, which can worsen depression and hinder treatment. If you have been told you snore excessively or move constantly throughout the night, ask your doctor whether you should have a formal sleep evaluation.

Control stress

Stress is a big player in depression. Control it before it controls you. Great stress-busting techniques include yoga, meditation, progressive relaxation and guided imagery. Whenever you're feeling like your stress is getting out of control, take a step back. Take a vacation from work, leave your kids with a babysitter, get help taking care of an ailing spouse—whatever you need to do to regroup. Consider whether certain obligations can be tabled. For example, having lunch every day with a very negative co-worker may be a tradition that ought to be put on indefinite hold while you are working to get better from depression.

Put yourself in a position to experience pleasure

Even when you doubt that you will able to get pleasure out of experiences because of your depression, allow yourself to do the things you used to enjoy before your depression took root. Take a picnic lunch in the park. See a new movie that you would have normally loved. Accept an invitation for dinner with good friends. Don't expect to fully enjoy these moments until your depression is treated, but by continuing to give yourself opportunities to experience pleasure, you will contribute to your recovery.

Release your emotions

When you're feeling stressed out or sad, let it out. Bottled-up grief and anger can ferment inside you until it finally explodes. Talk about your

---

BOX 6-5

Improve your sleep habits

Are you getting a good night's sleep? Restless nights can lead to moody days. Here are some tips to help you fall asleep more easily and rest well until morning.

- Go to bed at the same time each night and wake up at the same time each morning.

- Avoid napping, which perpetuates the cycle of poor nighttime sleep and daytime drowsiness.

- Relax before bed by taking a warm bath, listening to soothing music or meditating.

- Don't exercise or watch TV right before bed. Also avoid stimulants like sugar and caffeine within a few hours of bedtime. People who are particularly sensitive to caffeine might need to avoid caffeine-laden food and drinks, such as coffee, tea, cola and chocolate, after lunchtime.

- Avoid alcohol, which may make you feel tired at first but can make sleep less restful.

- Try not to use your bedroom for activities other than sleep (and sex). Pay bills and do work elsewhere if you can.

- Keep your bedroom quiet, dark and comfortably cool.

feelings to family members, friends or a therapist. Or, write down your thoughts in a journal.

Finally, don't get discouraged

Instead of punishing yourself for failing to recover from your depression quickly, reward yourself for all the improvements you have made.

When Is Emergency Help Needed?

Sometimes people sink so deeply into depression that they can no longer see any hope. To them, the only possible future is one that doesn't include them. These people begin to contemplate taking their own life.

Depression is one of the biggest risk factors for suicide. Any thoughts of hurting yourself are very serious. Get help right away by calling a friend, your doctor or the National Suicide Prevention Hotline at: 1-800-SUICIDE (1-800-784-2433) or 1-800-273-TALK (1-800-273-8255).

If someone close to you has depression, look for these symptoms of a possible suicide risk:

- Being obsessed with death, talking about it all the time
- Engaging in risky behaviors, like drinking and driving
- Putting their affairs in order, such as finalizing a Last Will and Testament or giving away treasured objects or pets
- Saying things like, "Everyone will be better off when I'm gone"
- Calling people to say goodbye
- Talking or writing about committing suicide

If you see any of these signs, encourage the person to get help. If you think a suicide attempt is imminent, call 911 or get other emergency assistance right away.

Relapse Prevention

One of the most important, yet most neglected aspects of depression treatment is preventing depression from returning. Relapse refers to the return of depression after a period of doing well. The term recurrence sometimes refers to a relapse that occurs late, after many months or years of stable mood and functioning (unlike relapses that occur within weeks or months of responding to depression treatment).

Most research has been directed at the initial treatment for depression rather than on maintaining health once the depression has resolved. Similarly, most doctors and patients are focused so intently on the goal of recovering from depression that the idea of preventing a relapse is almost an afterthought. Nevertheless, the statistics speak for themselves. Anyone who has had one episode of major depression has at least a 50 percent chance of experiencing another episode at some point in his or her life. Anyone who has had two or more episodes of depression, has had periods of depression that have lasted for years, has been hospitalized for depression, or has not fully recovered from a current episode of depression has an extremely high likelihood of relapse, even over the next 12 months. This means that for many people, depression is not simply an "episode," but a long-term disorder—like high blood pressure or diabetes—that requires long-term management.

You need to go into treatment with the expectation that you may have periods of improvement and periods in which your symptoms get worse. It is essential that you discuss relapse prevention the doctor or mental health professional who is treating your depression.

For most patients, identifying the warning signs that their depression is returning (such as becoming more isolated or not responding to emails and phone calls) can help nip a relapse in the bud. For many people, identifying triggers of past depression (such as a loss, move, disappointment or work stress) can also help them develop a treatment plan with their health care provider that reduces the likelihood of a full-blown relapse in the future.

Patients with severe depression or a history of relapses can benefit from staying on medications for several years and having regular mental health or primary care visits. For others, continued individual or group psychotherapy sessions at stressful times can help with treatment and monitoring. Participating in a self-help group like the Depression and Bipolar Support Alliance (see *Resources*, page 80) can be a very helpful form of support and education. For individuals with very severe depression that has required ECT, it may be worthwhile to consider having a series of once monthly "maintenance ECT" treatments.

Whatever treatments you consider for relapse prevention, it is crucial that you discuss them with your mental health care provider as part of your overall health care plan.

Healthy Steps

Here are a few other healthy steps can you take to improve your health and quality of life:

■ Work to build new social supports

■ Tackle recurrent sources of frustration in your career or home life

■ Achieve more healthy diet and exercise habits

■ Develop new hobbies

If you are going to successfully treat your depression and keep it under control for many years, your treatment must be part of an overall healthy lifestyle. There is no guarantee that depression won't come back. Even when you are doing everything right, depression can relapse. But by doing all the right things, you are more likely to bring your depression under control so you can get back to your life. ■

7 CONCLUSION

We hope that after reading this report, you'll have a much better understanding of depression—its causes, symptoms, prevalence and most importantly, how to get help when you or someone you know is experiencing persistent dark moods.

Depression can be one of the most isolating conditions. It makes people retreat from their friends, family, job and life as a whole. But when you realize just how many people have depression—almost 21 million people in America—you can't help but feel far less alone. Think about your friends, your neighbors and the people you work with. Many of them are going through or have gotten through exactly what you are experiencing right now.

Compare the symptoms you are experiencing against the checklist on page 38. If you check off several of these signs of depression, make an appointment with your primary care doctor or a mental health professional. Get diagnosed, and get started on your treatment now, so you can get back to your life and loved ones.

Know that there are many treatments for depression, and they do work. Medications, therapy and brain stimulation techniques have helped people just like you escape from their depression—often permanently. Researchers around the world are working hard to learn more about depression and its roots in the brain. What they are discovering is opening the doors to newer and potentially even better treatments in the years to come. ■

APPENDIX I: GLOSSARY

Adrenaline (epinephrine): A hormone and neurotransmitter that stimulates the heart, blood vessels and circulatory system.

Anhedonia: A common symptom of chronic depression characterized by the inability to feel pleasure.

Anxiolytics: Drugs used to treat anxiety. These are sometimes used for depression that has an anxiety component.

Antipsychotics: Drugs that are typically used to treat symptoms of psychosis, such as hallucinations and delusions, but that also sometimes play a role in the treatment of depression.

Antidepressants: Medications that improve mood and functioning in people with depression by regulating the levels of neurotransmitters in the brain.

Atypical depression: A type of depression that includes symptoms of overeating, oversleeping, sensitivity to rejection or criticism and the ability to temporarily respond to happy or positive events.

Axon: An extension that carries impulses from one nerve cell to another.

Baby blues: Normal feelings of sadness or being overwhelmed in the first days after bringing a baby home that rapidly diminish without treatment.

Bipolar disorder: A mental disorder in which the person experiences mood swings from mania to depression. Symptoms often include euphoria, irritability, high energy and activity, a reduced need for sleep, rapid thoughts and speech, a grandiose sense of one's talents or power and impulsive behaviors such as spending sprees or promiscuous sexual activity.

Borderline personality disorder: A psychiatric condition typically characterized by profound feelings of emptiness, unstable interpersonal relationships, self-destructive behaviors and suicidal tendencies.

Brain stem: The bundle of nerves at the base of the brain that allow the brain and body to communicate. The brainstem regulates basic functions such as sleep, arousal, breathing and heart rate.

Brain stimulation therapy: A treatment for depression that involves stimulating the brain or nervous system.

Cerebellum: The part of the brain related to movement, balance and emotion.

Cerebrum: The largest part of the brain, which is responsible for conscious mental processes such as thinking, learning and memory.

Clinical depression: Another term for major depression.

Cognitive behavioral therapy (CBT): A structured form of psychotherapy that helps people address the negative and often irrational thoughts and self-defeating behaviors that may cause or perpetuate their depression.

Concreteness training (CNT): A new form of therapy that focuses on teaching depressed people to think concretely instead of ruminate about and overgeneralize problems and negative thoughts.

Cortisol: A hormone that is involved with the body's stress response. In some, but not all people with depression, cortisol levels are elevated.

Deep brain stimulation: A technique that uses implanted electrodes to directly stimulate parts of the brain involved in mood.

Delusion: A symptom of psychosis in which a person has a belief, often bizarre, that has no basis in reality.

Dendrite: A branching structure that connects nerve cells to one another.

Dialectical behavior therapy: A type of psychotherapy that emphasizes acceptance and change.

Disruptive mood regulation disorder: A proposed type of depression that first manifests in childhood characterized by an irritable mood punctuated with outbursts of temper.

Dopamine: A neurotransmitter that is involved with movement and is part of the brain's pleasure-reward center.

Double depression: The term used when dysthymia and major depression overlap.

Dual diagnosis: When a Substance Use Disorder such as alcohol or drug addiction co-occurs with another psychiatric disorder such as major depressive disorder or bipolar disorder.

Dysthymia: A type of depression in which symptoms are chronic (lasting at least two years) but generally less severe than those of major depression.

Electroconvulsive therapy (ECT): A depression treatment that passes a controlled electric current through the brain to produce seizures while the patient is asleep under anesthesia.

Epigenetics: The study of heritable changes in how genes function that occur without changing the actual sequence of DNA. These changes in the expression of genes may be induced by environmental or other factors.

Hallucination: A symptom of psychosis characterized by hearing or seeing things that are not there.

Hippocampus: A structure in the brain that is involved in short-term and long-term memory.

Hypomania: A milder form of mania.

Hypothalamic-pituitary-adrenal axis (HPA axis): A complex system that is involved in the body's response to stress.

Hypothyroidism: A condition in which the thyroid gland becomes underactive. Hypothyroidism sometimes causes symptoms that mimic depression, such as low energy, weight gain or difficulty thinking or remembering.

Interpersonal therapy: A type of psychotherapy that addresses the conflicts, communication issues and other relationship problems that can impact depression.

Leptin: A hormone produced by human fat cells that may play a role in depression.

Magnetic resonance imaging (MRI): An imaging technique that uses magnetic fields instead of x-rays to visualize the structures and functions of the body, including the brain.

Major depression: Depressed or irritable mood, feelings of worthlessness and guilt and other symptoms such as sleep, appetite and concentration changes that last for more than two weeks and are significant enough to interfere with a person's life.

Mania: A state experienced by people with bipolar disorder characterized by great euphoria, overactivity, decreased need for sleep, irritability, impulsivity, racing thoughts and rapid speech and sometimes hallucinations and delusions.

Mixed episode: A period in which individuals with bipolar disorder experience symptoms of both mania and depression at the same time, such as intense sadness combined with rapid thoughts and increased energy.

Mood stabilizer: A type of drug that helps regulate the pattern of extremely high and low moods experienced by people with bipolar disorder such as lithium, valproic acid, lamotrigene or certain antipsychotic medications.

Monoamine oxidase inhibitors (MAOIs): A class of antidepressant drugs that work by preventing the enzyme monoamine oxidase from breaking down the neurotransmitters serotonin, norepinephrine and dopamine in the brain.

Neurons: Specialized cells of the nervous system that transmit electrical and chemical messages throughout the brain and body.

Neurotransmitters: Chemical messengers that are released by one neuron and activate or inhibit the activity of other neurons.

Norepinephrine: A neurotransmitter and hormone that is involved in the body's "fight-or-flight" arousal response, as well as in regulating mood.

Omega-3 fatty acids: A healthy form of fat found in fatty fish, flaxseeds and other foods that may play a role in staving off depression.

Postpartum depression: Depressed mood that occurs in the mother after the birth of her baby and lasts for more than two weeks after delivery. Unlike the "baby blues," which typically lift on their own within the first days or weeks of a baby's arrival, postpartum depression is a serious illness that needs to be evaluated and treated.

Postpartum psychosis: Confusion, loss of reality and severe depression that can occur in the mother after childbirth. This is a medical emergency, because the mother can have thoughts about hurting herself or her baby.

Premenstrual dysmorphic disorder: A type of short-lived but recurrent depression that occurs during the premenstrual period and then diminishes or disappears as menses begin.

Psychiatrist: A medical doctor who treats depression and other mental disorders. Psychiatrists can prescribe medications and order laboratory tests such as blood tests or brain imaging. Psychiatrists also conduct talk therapy (psychotherapy) sessions or work with other colleagues (such as psychologists or social workers) who provide talk therapy.

Psychodynamic therapy: A form of treatment that seeks to identify the roots of depression and develop new insights about how they have contributed to a person's thoughts and behaviors.

Psychologist: A mental health professional who can diagnose and treat depression. In most states, psychologists are not licensed to prescribe medications. Instead, they specialize in providing talk therapy (psychotherapy). Some psychologists are also trained to do special forms of cognitive or educational testing. Psychologists usually have a master's or doctorate degree.

Psychotherapy: A treatment in which a therapist helps the patient talk through and try to find solutions to the issues that are causing depression. Several different types of talk therapies are conducted individually or in groups, such as cognitive behavioral therapy, interpersonal therapy and psychodynamic therapy.

Psychotic depression: A form of depression in which a person hallucinates, has false beliefs and loses touch with reality. Often treatment for psychotic depression involves hospitalization and may include antipsychotic or antidepressant medication or electroconvulsive therapy.

Receptor: A structure on the neuron that receives a chemical signal.

Recurrence: The return of depression following a long period, usually years, of doing well.

Relapse: The return of depression following a relatively short period, usually weeks or months, of doing well.

Remission: The full return of normal moods and functioning following an episode of depression.

Seasonal affective disorder (SAD): Symptoms of depression that regularly occur with the change in seasons, and persist through the season (typically winter).

Selective serotonin reuptake inhibitors (SSRIs): A class of antidepressants that treat depression by blocking the reuptake of serotonin, making more of the neurotransmitter available to the brain.

Serotonin: A neurotransmitter that is involved with mood and sleep.

Serotonin and norepinephrine reuptake inhibitors (SNRIs): A class of antidepressants that treat depression by blocking the reuptake of both serotonin and norepinephrine, making more of these neurotransmitters available to the brain.

Social Worker: A clinician with a graduate degree and license in social work who may provide individual or group psychotherapy or may provide case management within a treatment team.

Substance-induced depression: A type of depression brought on by taking medications or other drugs.

Subthreshold hypomania: A type of hypomania experienced by some people with depression that is too mild to be officially diagnosed as hypomania.

Synapse: The tiny gap between nerve cells across which nerve signals pass.

Thyroid gland: The butterfly-shaped gland in the neck that produces the hormones that regulate growth, development, and energy use.

Transcranial direct current stimulation (tDCS): A brain stimulation treatment for depression that uses electrodes placed on the scalp to deliver a mild current to the front portion of the brain.

Transcranial magnetic stimulation (TMS): A non-invasive therapy that has been approved by the Food and Drug Administration for treating depression. TMS relieves depression by using magnetic fields to send weak electrical currents into the brain.

Treatment-resistant depression: Depression that does not respond to one or more courses of treatment (which most often involves taking a full dose of an antidepressant for at least eight to 12 weeks).

Tricyclic antidepressants: An older class of antidepressant that improves mood by increasing levels of serotonin and norepinephrine in the brain.

Trigeminal nerve stimulation: A treatment originally designed for epilepsy but that is also showing promise in depression that involves delivering a mild electric current the trigeminal nerve in the face.

Vagus nerve stimulation (VNS): A therapy approved by the Food and Drug Administration for treatment-resistant depression. VNS involves implanting a device called a pulse generator in the chest, which sends electrical impulses to the vagus nerve in the brain. These signals affect parts of the brain that regulate mood.

APPENDIX II: RESOURCES

For general information about depression, contact the following organizations:

**American Academy of Child
and Adolescent Psychiatry**
3615 Wisconsin Avenue, N.W.
Washington, D.C. 20016-3007
(202) 966-7300
www.aacap.org

American Foundation for Suicide Prevention
120 Wall Street, 22nd Floor
New York, NY 10005
(888) 333-AFSP (2377)
www.afsp.org

American Psychiatric Association
1000 Wilson Boulevard, Suite 1825
Arlington, VA 22209
(888) 35-PSYCH (77924)
www.psych.org

American Psychological Association
750 First Street NE
Washington, D.C. 20002-4242
(800) 374-2721 or (202) 336-5500
www.apa.org

American Society for Adolescent Psychiatry
P.O. Box 570218
Dallas, TX 75357-0218
(972) 613-0985
www.adolpsych.orgs

Depression and Bipolar Support Alliance
730 N. Franklin Street, Suite 501
Chicago, IL 60654-7225
(800) 826-3632
www.dbsalliance.org

**Massachusetts General Hospital
Women's Mental Health Program**
www.womensmentalhealth.com

Mental Health America
2000 N. Beauregard Street, 6th Floor
Alexandria, VA 22311
(800) 969-6642
www.nmha.org

National Alliance on Mental Illness (NAMI)
3803 N. Fairfax Drive, Ste. 100
Arlington, VA 22203
(703) 524-7600
www.nami.org

**National Council for Community
Behavioral Healthcare**
1701 K Street NW, Suite 400
Washington, D.C. 20006
(202) 684-7457
www.thenationalcouncil.org

Moodbook
The National Network of Depression Centers
2929 Plymouth Road, Suite 300
Ann Arbor, MI 48105
(734) 332-3914
www.moodbook.nndc.org

National Institute of Mental Health
6001 Executive Blvd., Room 8184, MSC 9663
Bethesda, MD 20892-9663
(866) 615-6464
www.nimh.nih.gov

National Network of Depression Centers
www.nndc.org

National Suicide Prevention Lifeline
1-800-273-TALK (8255)
www.suicidepreventionlifeline.org

**Substance Abuse and Mental Health Services
Administration (SAMHSA)**
1 Choke Cherry Road
Rockville, MD 20857
(800) SAMHSA-7
If in distress, call: (800)-273-TALK (8255)
www.samhsa.gov

SAMHSA's Center for Mental Health Services Locator
store.samhsa.gov/mhlocator

SAMHSA's National Mental Health Information Center
800-789-2647 or 240-221-4021
healthfinder.gov/orgs/HR2480.htm